Don't ever let pain **define you**

" Erica Meloe is a miracle-worker. Whenever I pull a muscle in my back or neck, I drag myself into her office, and after just one session, I get enormous relief. I've recommended her to countless friends. "

Gretchen Rubin
Bestselling author of *The Happiness Project* and *The Four Tendencies*

" Several years ago, I suffered an acute injury which eventually became chronic. I had been out of work almost a year for an injury that should have taken six weeks to heal. I was passed to three different physical therapists because no one could figure out why I wasn't getting better, a process that was frustrating, disheartening, and downright depressing. I felt betrayed by my body and believed I'd never be able to walk without excruciating pain for the rest of my life. Finally, a dear friend recommended Erica to me. At the FIRST APPOINTMENT, I was able to do something I hadn't done for *two years*: stand on my toes! Erica's solid guidance, simple exercises, and whole body approach led to my return to full duty at work in *five weeks*. As a professional Broadway actress, I depend on my body to do everything from wearing twenty-five pounds of costumes while dancing to carrying groceries through the fast-paced streets of New York City. Erica's method gave me my body, my livelihood, and my spirit back. I cannot recommend her approach highly enough. Give yourself the gift of taking control of your recovery and healing your body NOW! "

Satomi Hofmann
Broadway, Film, and Television Actress

" I am a professional dancer who first came to Erica for a sacroiliac injury. I was performing in a production for a few years where I was asked to do repetitive, one-sided movement. It wreaked havoc on my body in more ways than one. Erica's approach to assessment is very unique, integrative, and thorough. She not only figured out the improper mechanics that resulted in my SI injury, but found the link to a host of other chronic injuries I had been dealing with. With excellent manual therapy and a clear exercise plan, Erica helped heal my body and come up with an effective preventative plan moving forward. I would highly recommend her to anyone! "

Sharon Milanese
Dancer and rehearsal director for the Lucinda Childs Dance Company

"Erica has completely changed my life. Before starting sessions with her I had seen seven doctors, been on and off crutches, and almost scheduled surgery to remove a bone from my foot as a last resort. Within a month of working with her, I was back dancing and feeling like myself again for the first time in a year. Erica is a master at understanding both the physical and psychological damage of injury. She has given me back confidence in my body and the ability to continue pursuing my dreams. Her patience and knowledge is unmatched, and without her I may never have been able to recover."

Carrie Dickson
Dancer

"After unsuccessfully working with several different doctors, Erica got me on the road to recovery. Erica looked beyond my symptoms and conducted a holistic assessment of my posture and movements in order to discover the real source of my pain. Erica's diagnostic skills are superb. She then developed a treatment plan that included approaches for retraining my muscles. Without this sort of assessment and treatment plan, I am certain I would still be using a crutch or a cane to walk."

Maureen Massaro

"I've been working with Erica for over a decade now, and she is the best in the business. As an avid runner and a running coach, she is the first person I turn to when something isn't right with me or my clients. I initially sought Erica's help after a nagging ITB issue wouldn't go away. I had seen two different PTs before Erica, and neither of them offered the level of attention or expertise that Erica gave me. Within two months, I was pain-free and have been symptom-free ever since. A few years later, I returned to Erica for rehab on my achilles and my spine after two fluke injuries. Again, Erica's personal approach and commitment to my health were unbeatable. Unlike many PTs who walk you through the machines and sometimes only spend ten minutes with you, Erica is present the entire visit, and her style of manual therapy is very effective. Not to mention, she will teach you about the effectiveness of a little thing called preventative care. Thank you, Erica, for keeping me healthy!"

Jessica Green
RRCA Running Coach

" I was looking for a physiotherapist while living in the United States for a year, and I came across Erica. After suffering from undiagnosed pelvic girdle and low-back pain for approximately seven years, which prevented me from running and mobilizing pain-free, Erica was able to help me get back to running. I've seen multiple physiotherapists, osteopaths and chiropractors who were unable to place their finger on what was driving my pain. Erica's vast experience and detail-oriented assessment skills were able to correctly identify the root of my problems and get me back into my running shoes; for that, I am extremely grateful. It was an absolute pleasure working with Erica, and I recommend her to my friends suffering from persistent pain. "

Janelle Syring, BMR(PT)
Medical Student, McMaster University
Hamilton, Ontario, Canada

" My entire right shoulder girdle seemed to be out of alignment for over a year, causing me neck pain, preventing me from lifting weights, and even causing my right sterno-clavicular joint to protrude markedly. I had been seeing a well-regarded physical therapist for a year but without success; indeed, I got progressively worse. Then my trainer recommended Erica and within two months I was noticeably better; within four months I was 90 percent of normal. Erica really understands the human body, but can also translate that knowledge in a way that the layperson can understand, giving me simple exercises that I could do on my own. Since then, I have seen Erica for other ailments that seem to come more frequently with age, and have always come away "fixed." I have recommended friends to her on multiple occasions, who have universally thanked me for the life-changing referral. "

Chris Wilson
Partner, Stonehill Capital

Erica's approach to physical therapy is exceptional for this simple reason: She treats the person, not the injury. Her approach to every injury I have had has been unique and specific to my body. I've constantly been surprised at where Erica found the root causes of various shoulder and knee ailments (they weren't the knees or shoulders per se), and every time she treated those areas I was able to heal effectively. Even more remarkable was that, despite tears to my ACL and MCL, she managed to treat me so that I didn't need surgery and eventually returned to better than full strength. I think my basketball game actually got better after the injury and rehab. The true strength of Erica's approach is her ability to listen. She listened to what I was experiencing and made sure she took that into account. Even more remarkable, through treatment I could feel her listening to my body. Every muscle shift, creak, and crack gave her more information on finding the root cause of the pain, which was not always the site of an injury. Through experimentation and exploration, she uncovered the true source of my pain and likely culprits of my injury in the first place. In the long run, that's why I haven't had to go back to her frequently.

Jeffrey Golde
Golde Consulting
Adjunct Professor of Management, Columbia Business School

Having had several knee surgeries, and back and shoulder injuries, I have seen five physical therapists over the last ten years. I can say Erica is the best physical therapist I have encountered. She looks at your pain in a very holistic way, treating the whole body, not just the affected area. Working with her has kept me on the golf course and tennis courts. Erica spends the session working with you alone. You are not one of many patients lying on a table in the middle of a gym.

Sandra Coughlin

" I've had many injuries, several orthopedic surgeries, and I was in pain every day for years. I have worked with numerous physical therapists, chiropractors, acupuncturists and they have helped, but the pain and discomfort always came back in a few days. Since I've started working one-on-one with Erica Meloe, my body is more relaxed, in better alignment, and I have little to no pain.

" Erica searched for the core cause of my problem and almost immediately my body started to relax, release, realign, and respond to her therapeutic techniques. She explains what she is doing, and you work in partnership with her. Erica is gentle, comforting, knowledgeable, and skilled in her work. I haven't felt this good in years. "

Hermes Torres

why do I hurt?

Discover the surprising connections
that cause physical pain—
and what to do about them

Erica Meloe

PT, MBA, OCS, COMT

Foreword by Robert E. Rubin,
former Secretary of the Treasury

Why Do I Hurt?
Discover the Surprising Connections That Cause
Physical Pain—and What to Do About Them

Paperback ISBN: 978-0-9989939-0-4
Hardcover ISBN: 978-0-9989939-2-8
Printed in the United States of America

In loving memory of my parents
Basil and Torleif Meloe,
my guardian angels.

And for Brooke, my ever-faithful book buddy.
Declare your superpowers, girl!

Acknowledgments

Where do I start?

I am deeply honored by all the physical therapy rock stars who have entrusted me with their bodies, their minds, and their hearts. You all know who you are. My patients, I honor and love you, forever and ever.

To the people who have entrusted me with their stories in this book, you have made me rise up. I am truly thankful.

I honor my sister, Margaret, who has the guts to tell it like it is, no holds barred, and certainly the truth. So grateful for you.

I honor Lloyd, who digs deep and gets to what really matters. And isn't that the truth?

I love you, Brooke, to whom this book is dedicated to. Rise up, sister, and claim your truth. It is now or never, sweetheart.

And to Bob Rubin, who has written this foreword. I honor your honesty, your eloquence, your curiosity, and your trust.

To Beth Lottig, editor extraordinaire! Above and beyond, girlfriend, seriously. The top of your profession, to say the least. Not only do you understand writers, you empower them to a level like no other! I TRUST you, without doubt, to eternity.

To Frances Pharr, love your design eloquence, your sweetness and your extraordinary talent!! Your talents are at the TOP of your profession, truly! You propelled me to the finish line. Love you for that. You rock!!! #graphicdesignextraordinaire

To Debra Russell, where do I start? I cannot even begin to write to what extent you have helped me over the years. You really get it, don't you? You have an extraordinary gift of pulling the best out of people. You are truly superb and that is an understatement.

To Christine Gallagher, who just always does the right thing at the right time. The epitome of a person who knows what it really means to rise up to the top and certainly much more. You give of yourself endlessly.

To Jane Austen, LOVE always. You are always my escape. When people continue to talk about you HUNDREDS of years after death, you know you have a legacy.

To Tony Robbins, listening to your Personal Power tapes gave me the courage to leave Wall Street!

To my fellow physical therapists, you all know your value and what our future holds. Let's make a power grab like no other! Our patients are counting on us. Stand up for what you are worth. #donotholdback

To Erika, "Jenson" Smith. Holy Smokes!! You are THE BEST!!!! Future Emmy, Golden Globes, SAG, and OSCAR winner! Your production, direction, and writing exemplifies your true talent. Love you!!! Your absolutely graceful poses for this book make this extraordinary. You are truly a talent, bar none.

To Mom and Dad, I have tears in my eyes, every time I think of you. EVERY day I think of how you shaped me, how you would be proud of everything, your daughters and your granddaughter, Brooke, have done. Legacy is where it is at.

To Diane Lee and LJ Lee, who taught me how to evaluate and treat like a real physio. I honor your boldness, your compassion, and your grit to what really matters. You have made me rise up. Truly a game changer, to say the least.

X O X O
Erica

Table Of Contents

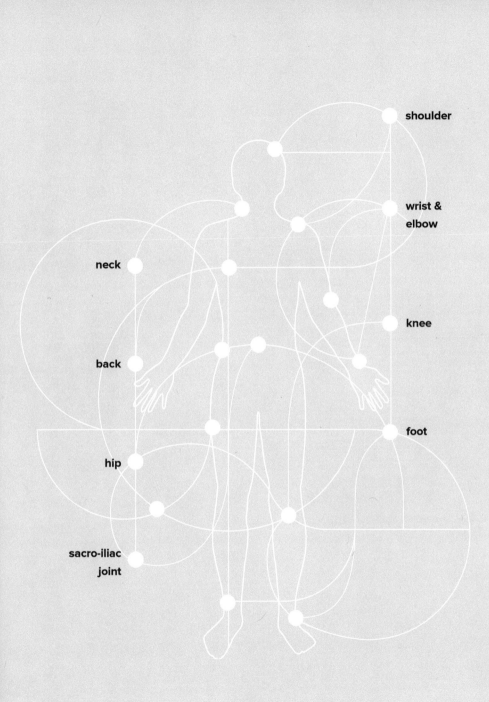

shoulder

wrist &
elbow

neck

knee

back

hip

foot

sacro-iliac
joint

Foreword

I first picked up a fly rod about thirty-five years ago, and I've been addicted to every aspect of fly fishing ever since—reading the water, casting, managing the line, and setting the hook, despite how often I mess it up. I've had the opportunity to cast a fly in some of the wondrous waters of the world, from the bonefish flats of the Bahamas to the rivers and spring creeks of Montana to the Atlantic salmon waters of Canada.

About ten years ago, I was fly fishing in Montana and did something that caused me tremendous pain. It affected me a lot, and was very limiting. No one could figure out what the issue was or, more importantly, how to make the pain go away. I was examined by distinguished doctors at distinguished hospitals. I had MRIs. The doctors catalogued a long list of potential problems. "Maybe you need a spinal fusion," one mused.

At the same time, I consulted my physical therapist, Erica Meloe. Erica diagnosed the problem as soft tissue. "I can feel it in my hands," she said. "And it's not difficult to deal with."

My doctors were dismissive. "She's a PT," they said. "What does she know?"

I'll tell you what Erica knew: She knew what was wrong and how to make the pain go away. That's what she did for me, and I'm forever grateful.

With this book, Erica shares her problem-solving, can-do approach to physical therapy, as well as her experienced view that all parts of the body are connected and that your pain can come from unexpected places. She dispels misperceptions about the profession, and gives you the information you need to find the PT that's right for you. Chronic pain affects more people than diabetes, heart disease, and cancer combined; that's why we need people like Erica more than ever. The book is not only instructive—with helpful case studies from her decades at the highest levels of the field—it's also an interesting and fun read. And that's unsurprising, because those are the traits that contribute to Erica being so successful at what she does: She's focused, effective, and a joy to work with.

Erica worked for some years in finance after receiving her MBA from the NYU Stern School of Business, and then she decided that she wanted to more directly help people. And I am grateful that she made that decision, because, thanks to her, I have many more years of fly fishing ahead of me.

Robert E. Rubin
Former Secretary of the Treasury

Movement is your **heart** and **soul**

Are you ready to discover
why you hurt?

What is this book about?

This book is about helping save people from suffering unnecessary persistent pain by providing them with the knowledge and resources that put them back in control of their own body.

Why did I write this book and what should I expect?

I always wanted to read a book like this, actually. As a patient, student, and a practicing clinician, I was starved for case studies and real-life examples of how other people were resolving their pain issues. I love to read stories, and getting a patient's history and their eventual treatment is the best story of all. You get to hear the whole story, and that's what makes case histories so interesting and relevant to my profession. As a matter of fact, the stories contained in this book provide the reader, patient, clinician, and researcher with much-needed information revealing other potential sources of typical pain patterns.

My hope is that this book will both inform and enlighten you as the reader and motivate you to advocate for yourself. I designed each chapter as part of a toolkit, meant to empower you to solve your own pain issues and help you discover the source of why you are not moving the way you want to.

To further reinforce the idea that we treat the cause of your problem and not just the symptoms, examples of creative and integrative treatment ideas are presented at the end of each chapter. These pages are highlighted in Tiffany Blue. You can refer to these treatment plans as needed, subsequent to your initial reading of the main body of the book.

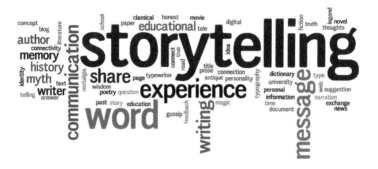

Truthfully, I got fed up with the misguided reputation that the physical therapy profession has in the eyes of the consumer, the medical community, and the government.

I use the term physiotherapy and physical therapy (PT), as well as physiotherapist and physical therapist, interchangeably throughout the book. The United States is the only country, as far as I know, who uses the term physical therapy. The rest of the world uses the term physiotherapy.[1]

Honestly, sifting through the myriad of information on the Internet can be mind-boggling for sure. People look for clarity and answers on the web when it comes to their health problems, and oftentimes they end up confused and scared. Talk about ramping up the nervous system. Whew!

I know a thing or two about a ramped-up nervous system. After all, I sat on a trading floor for ten years with neck and back pain with no one able to help me resolve it. After graduating from NYU Stern School of Business with my MBA, I took a position at an international investment bank in their international fixed income research department, where I sat all day.

---

1   Physical therapy (PT), also known as physiotherapy, is a primary care specialty in Western medicine that uses principles of bio-mechanics, kinesiology, the nervous system, manual therapy, exercise therapy, and various other physical therapies, which remediate impairments, promote mobility, function, and quality of life. This is done through examination, diagnosis, prognosis, and physical intervention. In addition to clinical practice, other activities encompassed in the physical therapy profession include research, education, consultation, and administration. Physical therapy services may be provided as primary care treatment.

Shortly thereafter, I moved to the trading floor, trading and selling international bonds and their derivatives. Even more sitting, more phone work, and more stress.

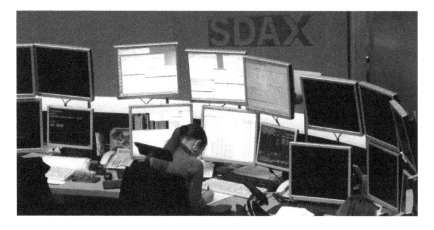

After a successful decade of problem-solving with clients on trading strategies and portfolio allocations, I decided to use those same skills in the field of physical therapy to help alleviate my patients' pain through a unique problem-solving approach.

And I got rid of my back and leg pain.

Back to why I wanted to write this book ...

- I want you to realize there could be other sources to your problem other than where your symptoms manifest.
- I want you to know that I understand the experience and frustration of persistent pain.
- I want you to understand that you are unique and what works for someone else may not work for you.
- I want to educate you, the patient and consumer, about potential causes of your pain.
- I want you to understand that just because you have back pain and look up exercises for your low-back, they have the potential to make you worse or at the very least not help you if the back is not the source of the problem.
- I want you to embrace the idea that physiotherapy should be your first line of defense for musculoskeletal disorders.

- I want you to understand that not all physical/physio therapists are alike.
- I want you to understand the unique clinical reasoning process that physical therapists employ to diagnose patients.
- I want you to learn how to advocate for yourself.
- I want to give you HOPE that it can get better.
- I want you to realize that there could be other possible sources potentially causing your pain.
- I want to encourage you to *not give up*, as I am sure there is another solution.

We will figure it out together. Let's get off the opioids and move on to getting yourself pain-free.

I understand that pain is depressing; it is cruel and unkind. It is also unforgiving at times. Pain appears when you least expect it and won't go away when you want it to go. However, if you think about your pain all day, it will make you worse. Research shows that the more you think about pain, the worse it becomes.[2]

" Let's get off the opioids and move on to getting yourself pain-free. "

You wake up in the morning and can't move.
You can't stand up straight.
You can't put your foot on the ground because your heel hurts.
You have a migraine because you were grinding your teeth all night.
You can't walk down the street because of your hip pain.
You can't even step up onto a curb because your hip hurts.
Stairs just about kill you because they hurt your knee.
Sitting at your desk all day bothers your back.
You can't go for a run because your ankle is sore.
You can't play golf because your elbow hurts.
You can't walk through an airport because your hamstring aches.
You can't reach across to turn the radio off in the morning because your shoulder is locked up and you have radiating pain down your arm.
And to top it all off, you throw your back out after hitting a tennis ball, and you've played tennis all your life.

---

2   Butler, David; Moseley, Lorimer. *Explain Pain*. NOI Group: 2013.

Do any of these sound familiar?

They are certainly familiar to me. I just described the many injuries I have experienced over the years, with varied causes, and I am sure I left a few out. Some were really ridiculous, like reaching over to turn off my radiator; others were not that benign.

I had a massage therapist drill her elbow into my shoulder blade, and then I could not move my arm the next day. Ouch. I love massage therapists—just not that one.

One of my patients started to faint, and I went to grab her so she would not fall to the floor. I tore my hamstring in the process, and then I went to the floor. That was a bad one. Took me out for months.

When I was in Arizona one Christmas, I hit with one of the pros at the resort where I was staying. I had played competitive tennis when I was younger, so I really got into it. The next morning I could barely stand up straight and then had to get on a flight back to New York. The flight was three hours delayed, which we found out once we got on the plane and then had to deplane. You can imagine how that must have felt.

One of the worst and most chronic ones is waking up every day with a headache and sometimes a full-blown migraine. Now that's a nice way to start your day, right? Feeling like a Mack truck has hit you in the face.

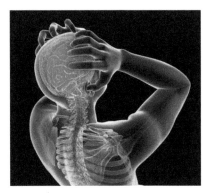

When you sustain an injury, you want help. It seems that everyone is a doctor when you relate your story. They all give you advice—some you take and some you don't. You're desperate to feel better. I get it.

But you are special. You are unique. What worked for your friend may not work for you. What worked for someone on the Internet may not work for you, and you do not even know that person!

My purpose in writing this book is to educate you the patient, the consumer, about the potential of other areas of your body—areas you may not even have considered—that could be causing your pain. If you have not gotten better with treatment done to the symptomatic part, then PLEASE consider that there could be other potential sources to your problem.

I hope this book will convince you that good physical therapy and seeing a *good* physical therapist should be your first line of defense for musculoskeletal disorders. If you do not get the results that you want, then I give you permission to advocate for yourself, and see another physical therapist; not a chiropractor, not an osteopath, not a massage therapist, not a personal trainer, not an acupuncturist, but another physical therapist, and a good one at that.

My goal is not to disparage those professions but to encourage you to allow physiotherapy to work for you. I appreciate all of the contributions that other professions make to our health care system. However, the superior clinical reasoning process physical therapists utilize is what sets us apart from the rest of the allied health professions. *We are the experts in movement.*

In my clinical practice, I often hear from patients that all PTs are alike. "When you've been to one, they are all the same." That both saddens and irritates me every time I hear it.

I also believe that other allied health professionals have a disjointed view of our profession. Case in point, a patient reschedules her appointments because her doctor wants her to take it easy, even after the patient tells the physician that she is not doing anything strenuous in therapy. As a matter of fact, she is lying on the table having certain muscles and joints released and getting some tape on her shoulders. I mean, really? Does that sound strenuous? She exerted more effort getting out of bed that day.

This book is *an excellent introduction* for patients and practitioners as to other potential sources of pain. It describes a unique clinical reasoning process and educates others as to how a structure or process far away from the symptom could be causing a person's pain.

Do you have pain or dysfunction that is unresolved?

Are you frustrated that you are not getting the results that you expected?

Do you want to get to the bottom of it all?

This book is *also a guide* to making sure that you have found the right physical therapist, as well as the right physical therapy, for you. A good **PT** who gets it. It is vitally important to see a practitioner who gets your full story and listens to you.

I am sure many of you out there who have picked up this book have done so for a reason. You may have persistent pain or pain that just won't go away despite having been treated for it, or maybe you are looking for another more holistic approach.

Persistent pain is a significant health problem.

According to the Institute of Medicine, chronic pain in the United States affects more people than diabetes, heart disease, and cancer combined. It is estimated that the economic cost of chronic pain in the United States is between $560 and $635 billion dollars.[3] And pain can kill. There are several reports of suicides relating to chronic pain.[4] I recently saw an alarming statistic stating that only 10 percent of patients who saw a primary care doctor for low-back pain were referred to physiotherapy. What happened to the other 90 percent? Given drugs and sent on their way?[5] What do you think of those statistics? Pretty daunting, right?

Persistent pain is a significant health problem.

When you're in pain, you want a diagnosis, you want to tell your story to someone, you want to be heard, you want to move freely, and, above all, you want to heal and move forward.

However, relief of pain does not guarantee full function. And full function does not mean that you are pain-free.

---

3   Gaskin, Darrell J.; Richard, Patrick, "The Economic Costs of Pain in the United States," *Journal of Pain*, Vol 13, Issue 8, 715-724. August 2012.

4   Institute of Medicine Report from the Committee on Advancing Pain Research, Care, and Education: *Relieving Pain in America, A Blueprint for Transforming Prevention, Care, Education and Research.* The National Academies Press, 2011.http://books.nap.edu/openbook.php?record_id=13172&page=1.

5   Zheng P1, Kao MC, Karayannis NV, Smuck M., "Stagnant Physical Therapy Referral Rates Alongside Rising Opioid Prescription Rates in Patients With Low-back Pain in the United States," Spine, 42(9), 670-674: May 1, 2017.

I am so grateful that I am part of a profession that helps heal people. Physical therapists are the consummate experts in movement dysfunction—hands down.

The problem in our society today is that we treat the symptoms, not the sources. In fact, when you take a whole-body approach, including your nervous system, your musculoskeletal system, your visceral system, etc. you have an INTEGRATED approach to care.

Isn't that what you want?

Believe or not, your symptom tells us nothing about the causes of your problem. You have back pain? A lot of people have back pain, but trust me—they do not have the same cause.

I am not averse to treating the symptom, but oftentimes it is secondary—especially when the problem is a persistent one. If you have had the symptom long enough, then, more often than not, some treatment to the area is necessary. However, it is important to note that treatment to the symptomatic area alone will not provide you with total relief, and the pain may eventually come back.

This is also true for multiple symptoms. They are usually all connected. The concept of the kinetic chain originated in 1875 when a mechanical engineer, Franz Reuleaux (1829–1905)—often called the father of kinematics—proposed that if a series of overlapping segments were connected via pin joints, these interlocking joints would create a system that would allow the movement of one joint to affect the movement of another joint within the kinetic link.[6,7]

A *kinetic chain* is the notion that these joints and segments have an effect on one another during movement; when one is in motion, it creates a *chain* of events that affects the movement of neighboring joints, segments, and systems, which include the nervous system.

In short, every action within our body creates a ripple effect across the whole kinetic chain, and that includes our heart and brain. They are part

---

6   Reuleaux, Franz. *Kinematics of Machinery*. Dover Publications: 2012.

7   Moon, Francis. "Franz Reuleaux: Contributions to 19th Century Kinematics and Theory of Machines." Cornell Library Technical Reports and Papers: 2002.

of a system that is called YOU.

You can see that even though people may have the same symptom, the treatment SHOULD be different. As people, we are so varied and diverse; don't we deserve a uniquely guided approach to our health care? The answer is *yes*.

An integrated approach is what is called for in order to address the whole person and bring about healing and lasting relief from pain.

In the pages of this book, you will discover, via some really interesting stories, the possibility of other areas of your body that could potentially be causing your symptoms. Additionally, you will learn what good physical therapy is and does, what makes it unique among the allied health professions, how you can find the right PT for you, and how others have found relief from persistent pain through physiotherapy.

You don't have to live with pain. Let's take a leap together and get you one step closer to living pain-free.

Why Physiotherapy?

Because it works, that's why.

Good physiotherapists excel in the clinical reasoning process. We are EXPERTS in movement analysis, and we can diagnose movement issues like no other health professional. And we offer the most holistic approach around.[8]

We excel at restoring movement, bar none. We should be the practitioner of choice when it comes to you, the consumer, accessing us for musculoskeletal disorders—whether it be for preventing an injury, general wellness, or a chronic pain problem that has not resolved.

---

8   Physical Therapist Practice and the Human Movement System. An American Physical Therapy Association White Paper. Alexandria, VA: American Physical Therapy Association; 2015.

" Everyone should get an annual movement exam. "

As a matter of fact, I think that everyone should get an annual movement exam. Just like getting your teeth cleaned and getting your annual physical, having a physical therapist assess you from a movement standpoint is key to keeping you at optimal performance.

Physical therapists are life span practitioners.

I'll write it again: *We are life span practitioners.*

In addition to being life span practitioners, PTs should be considered the first line in prevention when it comes to musculoskeletal issues. Not sure what that means? Consider the following questions.

- Do you want to start a new sport and are afraid you'll get injured?

- Do you want to return to a sport after a long period of absence?

- Is there a walking or running program you want to begin?

- Are you going on vacation and afraid your feet will hurt after walking all over the place?

- Have you just had a baby and are afraid to resume or start an exercise program?

- Has that old ankle sprain acted up right before your hiking vacation?

These are just some of the questions that a physical therapist will help you answer. Everyone—from corporate executives to elite athletes—are vulnerable to musculoskeletal issues at some point in their lives, and physiotherapists are ready to serve as the first line of defense for those whole-body issues.

In addition, our assessments encompass all the systems of the body, including the brain. Emotional and cognitive issues are very important factors in pain behavior, and a health care practitioner that does not take that into account is missing an important piece to your puzzle.

It is a well-known fact that persistent pain itself alters brain activity, which suggests that controlling pain becomes increasingly difficult as pain becomes more persistent.[9]

Health care is changing and consumers are more discerning when it comes to choosing a health care practitioner. They want value for their hard-earned money. Physical therapists offer better value than anyone else.

One of the pioneers of physical therapy once said, "I want physical therapists to take back exercise." I would go even further and add my own two cents to say, "I want physical therapists to own the realm of rehabbing musculoskeletal disorders, from diagnosis to discharge."

And discharge does not mean the end of treatment. Just because you have ended current treatment with your physical therapist does not mean that you are literally discharged. Does your dentist discharge you? Does your primary care physician discharge you? Continuing communication with your physical therapist is very important across your life span, especially as you get older and want to remain active.

Is the Physiotherapist In?

Oftentimes, patients tell me that they had to wait weeks to see their physician. Unfortunately, that is the case in our current health care system. Lengthy waits to get a doctor's appointment have become the norm in many parts of American medicine.[10] But why wait when you can see a physical therapist without a referral?

That is called direct access[11] in my words. In your words, that is called help, being seen, not having to wait, being given a diagnosis, taking the next step, moving forward ... however you want to name it.

Direct access—what's that?

---

9   Gifford, Louis. Topical Issues in Pain 3: Sympathetic nervous system and pain; Pain management; Clinical effectiveness. *Physiotherapy Pain Association*: 2013.

10   Rosenthal, Elisabeth. "The Health Care Waiting Game." *New York Times Sunday Review, News Analysis*. July 5, 2014. http://www.nytimes.com/2014/07/06/sunday-review/long-waits-for-doctors-appointments-have-become-the-norm.html?_r=0.

11   "Levels of Patient Access to Physical Therapist Services in the States." American Physical Therapy Association (APTA), May 2016, www.apta.org/uploadedFiles/APTAorg/Advocacy/State/Issues/Direct_Access/DirectAccessbyState.pdf

Direct access is a term used in many states to indicate that you as a consumer can access a PT's services without a doctor's prescription. For example, in my state of New York, we have limited direct access. As of this writing, that means that you can see me for thirty days or ten visits, whichever comes sooner, before you need a doctor's prescription.

As of 2016, all fifty states, the District of Columbia, and the US Virgin Islands allow patients to seek some level of care from a licensed physical therapist without a prescription or referral from a physician.[12]

This is EXTREMELY IMPORTANT, because it can take weeks before you are able to get an appointment with a physician. In the interim, you can directly access a PT, who will be able to assess, diagnose, and treat you. If we feel you need a referral to an MD, we will send you.

> **The irony is that we worked long and hard to get direct access and no one knows about it.**

For example, I had a patient some years ago now who came in to see me with complaints of swelling in his ankle. He had taken some time off to go traveling and did not know why his ankle was so swollen.

I examined him and believed that his swelling was not really swelling. It did not appear like a swollen ankle would appear. It felt strange. I referred him out to a physician I know. To make a long story short, he had a tumor in his ankle, which required extensive surgery. Thankfully, he is doing fine today.

I think one of the major hurdles in my field is that the average consumer does not know that they can access physical therapists directly. The irony is that we worked long and hard to get direct access and no one knows about it.

Where do I go? Can I see anyone I want?

Yes, you can see any physical therapist you want. If you are referred by a physician, for example, to a specific PT, and you want to go somewhere else because of a prior relationship or you've heard that the person

---

12   Please note: Direct Access Laws vary from state to state; please check with your local physical therapist as to whether or not you need a referral for PT. Direct Access also varies under Medicare. Please see footnote 11 on page 11 for a PDF download from the APTA.

is exceptional, you have the freedom of choice to go wherever you please. There is no hard and fast rule here. YOU GO WHERE YOU WANT.

Our patients are our best referral sources. "We depend on your word of mouth. Thank you for spreading the word." I love that saying! In fact, my email signature reads: "The highest compliment my patients can give me is to recommend me to a friend." I truly believe that.

Once they find a physical therapist, one of the first questions most people ask is, "Do you take my insurance?" This is not a book about the different health care options, but I will briefly tell you the difference between in-network and out-of-network here in the United States.

In-network means that the provider is contracted with the insurance company and provides care for a specific negotiated fee; they are in your network, so to speak.

> " At the end of the day, you go where you want to go. You go where you have the best chance of feeling better ... literally. "

Out-of-network means that the provider has not contracted with the insurance company. My practice is out-of-network and cash-based. In order to give the high quality care that YOU deserve, we MUST adhere to that business model.

For further information on your benefits, please check with your health insurance company and ask about your out-of-network PT benefits.

At the end of the day, you go where you want to go. You go where you have the best chance of feeling better ... literally. (Not where someone tells you that you have to go, not where your insurance company intimidates you into going, but where you want to go. Period. End of report.)

If you don't know where to go, then ask a friend, go online, educate and inform yourself ahead of time. Go on Instagram, Facebook, Twitter, or any of the social media sites and type in words like #lowbackpain if you have that. Type in #physicaltherapyhelp, #physiotherapyNYC #physicaltherapistnyc, etc. (you get the picture). Read the testimonials on their websites.

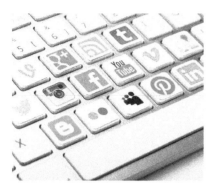

How do I interview a PT? What should I expect in a typical PT evaluation?

One often wonders the following when that first encounter is made with a medical professional:

Do I trust him/her?
Will they listen?
Can they give me a diagnosis?
Will I feel better?
What can I do to feel better?
Do they get me?
Am I on the right treatment plan?
Will they take my phone calls when I need something or ask a question?
Will they email me back?

Just because they are in a well-circulated newspaper, does that mean they are good? Absolutely not.

I always say, "Good people refer good people." When you see a medical professional—whether it be a physician, nurse, acupuncturist, physician's assistant (PA), occupational therapist (OT), or a physical therapist (PT)—you must leave their office believing you have seen a professional, or at the very least someone who has listened to you, understood your story, and will help you, advocate for you, listen to you, and work to HEAL you.

Patients want to be heard. I have been a patient many times, and the quality I most value in a health care practitioner is their ability to listen. It is amazing what you can glean from just listening to someone. Good communication between the provider and the patient lies in the ability of the provider to be present and attentive.[13]

Everyone has a story and, more often than not, telling their story is so therapeutic that afterwards they feel better. Have you ever had the experi-

---

13   Bensing, Jozien. "What Patients Want." Patient Education and Counseling, Vol. 90, Issue 3, pgs. 287-290. Elsevier Ireland Ltd: March 2013.

ence of unburdening yourself to someone, getting it all off your chest so to speak, and feeling lighter as a result? An immense relief envelops you.

The quality I most value in a health care practitioner is their ability to listen.

I believe that as physical therapists, the words that we speak to you are a vital, integral part of treatment. As such, they should be selected with care, just as we would select a treatment intervention, like joint mobilization or corrective exercise.

And your pain may not just be related to movement. Have you ever had a bad night's sleep and woke up the next morning with pain? Ever been sick with the flu and the knee that is always sore, is more sore? Research has shown that lack of good quality sleep affects not only how we feel mentally but also how we feel physically.[14] The immune system also plays a large role in how we feel in our bones, muscles, and joints.[15]

Poor "pain care," for lack of a better word, is a reality for many people. This happens EVERYWHERE, not just for the underserved population. Even elite athletes can struggle with getting good quality care for their injuries.

We know what we are used to, whether that is good or bad. However, when we explore beyond that, advocate for ourselves, and say, "Enough is enough!" and "I am sick and tired of feeling this way," then that is when we reach our true strength. It's that very strength that drives you to seek solutions for whatever is bothering you. Your problem could range from neck pain while sitting at your desk to constant back pain when you are competing in an Olympic gymnastics competition.

Knowledge is power and acting on that knowledge is even more powerful.

---

14   Schuch-Hofer, Sigrid, et al. "One night of total sleep deprivation promotes a state of generalized hyperalgesia: A surrogate pain model to study the relationship of insomnia and pain." Pain, Vol. 154, Issue 9, pgs. 1613-1621. Sept 2013.

15   Verma, Vivek, et al. "Nociception and role of Immune system in pain." Received 30 Nov 2014. Belgian Neurological Society: 2014.

What are the proper questions to ask before and during the first appointment?

When you call the office to make your first appointment and you get the insurance information out of the way, then you should ask the following questions:

How long are the evaluations?

In my office, evaluations are one hour. In my opinion, you cannot get a thorough evaluation and treatment done in thirty minutes, especially if you have had the problem for a long time. When an out-of-town patient comes in to see me, it can be up to two hours. Why? Because when that happens, they have likely seen multiple practitioners with little to no progress and they took the time to travel to see me.

Will I see the same therapist every time?

The answer should be yes. Barring vacations or illness, you should be with the same person the entire time—not with the PT for a few minutes and then an aide the rest of the time. Unless the therapist requests a second opinion from a colleague, your PT should not change, unless you request it.

This benefits you as well as the PT. Developing good relationships and a sense of trust is integral to the rehab process. We probably spend more time with you than any other health care professional, and the bond that you form with your PT is vital.

How long are the treatments?

Treatments are generally one hour but could range from thirty minutes to one hour. It depends on each unique patient and treatment situation. Some people need one hour while others need less. Keep in mind that we're talking one hour WITH the therapist, not fifteen minutes with the PT, fifteen minutes on a bike by yourself, and fifteen minutes on an electrical-stimulation machine followed by ice. You want quality time. Electrical stimulation does not replace quality time with a professional PT.

Again, physical therapists spend more time with patients than most other health practitioners. It is important to develop a trusting relationship with your PT.

What is considered good physical therapy?

The most important thing to consider when evaluating a physical therapist is how well they listened to your story in order to identify your unique issues. Did they spend ample time with you to give you a diagnosis? And by "ample time," I mean sixty minutes at least of listening to YOUR story about what brought you into their office, performing an in-depth assessment, and then giving you a thorough diagnosis as to what is causing your symptoms.

Most patients want to be heard. They *need* to be heard. It's cathartic for them to unburden themselves and tell their story of what hurts and how they want to get better. More often than not, they are even afraid to tell their own physicians their story in depth. They fear immobility, disability, and the loss of the active lifestyle they once had. When you are looking at someone holistically, as in treating the whole body, that means connecting with them *on an emotional level.*

An in-depth assessment includes looking at the whole body in a way that is meaningful to you. My expertise as a problem-solver is seeing people who have been elsewhere and have not gotten results. I don't know how many times patients of mine have told me that their prior practitioner told them they could only treat their knee, for example, because that is what is written on the prescription!

What you should expect from a good PT evaluation is a full-body assessment even if your problem is your foot and it's your hip that is causing the problem. The PT should assess your whole body. I had a patient who had a low-back problem, and I ended up treating her neck. She had numerous other interventions prior to seeing me, all treating the local area of pain, yet she did not get better. When I treated her neck, she did finally get better. Note: I will go into the details of her treatment in her story in the Low-back section of this book.

> **When you are looking at someone holistically, as in treating the whole body, that means connecting with them on an emotional level.**

The point of this is, if you have foot pain and a problem walking, then you should expect an analysis of your walking and all the relevant body components that need to move well in order for you to walk well, i.e., when you walk, your hips, pelvis, and mid-back need to rotate.

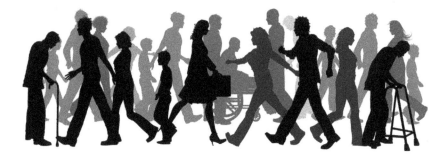

Just watch someone walk—our feet are not the only body parts moving. Some people walk with an arm swing, some don't. Some take longer steps while others do not. And if you need an assistive device like a cane or a walker, your gait is certainly different. If someone is just looking at the foot, they are doing you a disservice and may miss something important.

" What you should expect from a good PT evaluation is a full-body assessment. "

We are a movement profession as well as a hands-on profession. Watching someone move is extremely telling, and we should attempt to confirm our findings with our hands—kinesthetically. What you should expect is analysis of your movement as well as a hands-on evaluation and subsequent treatment.

For example, as I mentioned above, if your issue is pain with walking, then your PT will watch you walk. If your issue is running, then eventually running should be evaluated. During the first visit, that may be difficult because of space constraints, shoe apparel, etc. However, at some point, running should be assessed.

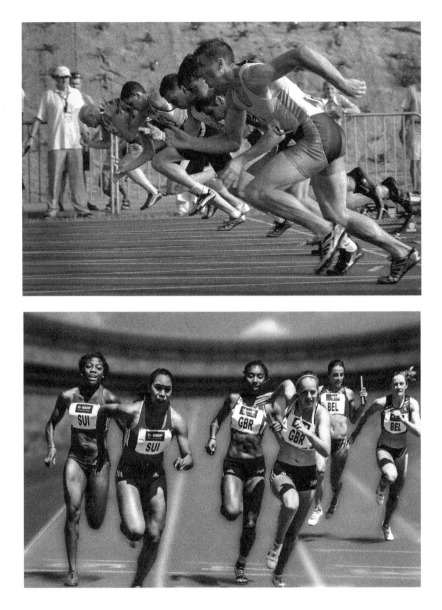

Initially, when a patient presents with problems running, I will look at a single leg balance, single leg mini squat, as well as rotation of the mid-back. After all, running is a one-legged activity, and we do not run with straight knees or a rigid back, as you can see above.

I evaluate these activities and determine visually and kinesthetically (with my hands)[16] to determine if the movement mechanics are optimal. Another example evaluation could be a patient who has a problem sitting, which is quite common. The assessment should include how you get to a seated posture (I look at the squat and a forward bend posture in this instance), as well as your actual sitting posture both in the clinic and in your office environment (this can be done via photos). I often find that it's what people do *while* they are sitting that's the root of the problem. Often, they are turned to the right or the left or they are reaching for their phone, etc.

Posture is a contentious issue in our society today. I believe that we can have many types of sitting postures that work well for us. It is the dominant one that's the game changer.

Patients sometimes say, "Well, I have been sitting that way for years." EXACTLY. You know the old saying: "You keep doing what you are doing, and you are going to get what you always got."

" This process IS the outcome. How you are assessed and evaluated is crucial to you feeling and moving better. "

Yet another example of an evaluation could involve a person who has an inability to reach behind their back. For example, they have trouble reaching for their seat belt, unhooking a bra, or putting their wallet in the back pocket. That particular move requires the synergistic action of multiple muscles and joints. In this case, we would then look at how that patient reaches their hand behind their back.

In my opinion, this kind of evaluation *validates* why you came in. Putting your hand behind your back, reaching overhead, sitting, walking, turning your head, whatever it is that brings on your symptoms—assessing that very movement justifies the reason you sought help.

This process IS the outcome. How you are assessed and evaluated is crucial to you feeling and moving better.

---

16   Kinesthetic: from the noun *kinesthesia*, which means the sensory perception of movement.

Furthermore, explaining why you hurt and helping you get a bigger and better grasp on understanding pain is very important. This is not only significant for acute pain but also for persistent pain—because pain of any sort does not serve a useful purpose long-term.[17]

What if they only use modalities, like ultrasound and electrical stimulation?

If you see a practitioner and all they do is put you on an electrical stimulation machine or have an aide do ultrasound, head for the door. That is NOT good physical therapy. There is no sound clinical reasoning going on here. In fact, there is no empirical evidence that ultrasound[18] or electrical stimulation provide adequate benefits to the patient long-term. I have not used an electrical stimulation machine or ultrasound for years now. Your valuable time can be spent doing other things to help you heal.

When is the right time for me to see another practitioner?

The right time is when you feel you are ready to move on. It may be to another PT or a referral back to your physician or a referral to another allied health practitioner. If you have been in physical therapy awhile and really have not improved a great deal, talk to your physical therapist.

The relationship is a two-way street and talking about other options is important and vital to your recovery. This assumes you are an active participant, meaning that you are listening to what your physiotherapist is telling you to do or not to do and adhering to your home program, what-ever that may be. I do not take home exercise programs lightly. They have to be realistic. Not five pages of ten exercises! Sometimes less is more. My best outcomes have been when my patients understand the "why" behind their home programs and the importance of sticking to them. And that also includes what not to do. Sometimes avoiding an activity or position for a while can be the key to getting you better.

---

17   Butler, David; Moseley, Lorimer. Explain Pain. NOI Group: 2013.

18   Ebadi, S; Nakhoustin, Ansari N.; Fallah E.; van Tulder, MW. Therapeutic ultrasound for chronic low-back pain. Cochrane Database of Systematic Reviews, The Cochrane Collaboration. John Wiley & Sons, LTD: 2014.

How long should I come to physical therapy?

That depends. Everyone heals differently and in their own time. If you have had surgery, there is a specific time frame involved for the tissue to heal, and that also is variable depending on YOU. You should respect your body's ability to heal itself. I tore my hamstring pretty badly two years ago, and it took a good five months at least for me to feel fully comfortable doing most activities.

Remember—everybody heals at their own rate.

Most people do not understand the level of commitment to the rehab process that they must adhere to after a surgical procedure. For example, I had a patient who had a rotator cuff repair and waited three months to start physical therapy, even though he had the go ahead to start from his physician. When he finally started coming, he came only once a week or once every other week, despite my advice to come two times a week. Obviously, that is not the most optimal scenario and would slow your recovery for sure.

Can't I manage this by myself if you give me exercises?

Generally not. Exercises are valuable and important in your program. However, if you have a mechanical issue that is contributing to your problem, then all the exercises in the world won't help you. You need an assessment from a physical therapist to determine if there is something else that needs to be done before you start an exercise program. What if you are exercising the wrong muscle group? Remember, if you exercise a body part that is not the cause of your problem, then you could worsen your symptoms and further delay your recovery.

What if I don't like someone touching me?

That's OK; touch is personal. When we touch someone, we invade your personal space. If you don't like that level of closeness, there are many other ways to help you heal. For example, research shows that the brain and mind play an enormous role in persistent pain syndromes (PPP).[19,20]

I once had a patient who had complaints of pain in her mid-back and was afraid to exercise at all—not just upper body work but all forms of exercise. When I told her that she was free to exercise and that she would be fine, she told me at our next meeting that all of her pain went away. *Words heal.*

Remember, words also hurt. Consider being told, "Based upon your MRI, you have a herniated disc and there is a fragment of the disc compressing a nerve in your spinal canal," or "Your MRI shows that you have a disc issue but that is not necessarily the cause of your problem. Many people have this and walk around pain-free." Same story, but different delivery. My all-time fave is "bone on bone." That is like a kiss of death to someone who has knee or hip pain. I was at a course recently, and David Butler, an international clinician, researcher, and educator, coined the term, "kisses of time." That sounds a hell of a lot better than bone on bone. Don't you think?

Talk about stressors. Pain is the universal stressor, and not understanding the "why" is one of the worst stressors of all.

As I stated previously, I believe that the words we speak to you as physical therapists are a vital part of treatment and, as such, should be selected with care. Just as we would carefully select a treatment intervention, like joint mobilization or corrective exercise, we should just as carefully select our words.

There is a great body of research out there on pain education, and it is an integral part of the treatment. If you don't want to open yourself up to someone touching you, that is okay. For starters, you can read *Explain Pain* by David Butler and Lorimer Moseley.[21] Sometimes, understanding is all you need.

---

19   Bushnell, M. Catherine; Ceko, Marta; Low, Lucie A. "Cognitive and emotional control of pain and its disruption in chronic pain." Nature, Vol 14, July 2013. Macmillan Publishers Limited: 2013.

20   Louw, Adriaan; Puentedura, Emilio J; Zimney, Kory; Schmidt, Stephen. "Know Pain, Know Gain? A Perspective on Pain Neuroscience Education in Physical Therapy." Journal of Orthopaedic & Sports Physical Therapy., Volume 46, No. 3, p. 131. March 2016.

21   Butler, David; Moseley, Lorimer. Explain Pain. NOI Group: 2013.

"Pain is the universal stressor, and not understanding the "why" is one of the worst stressors of all. "

Can I see my acupuncturist at the same time?

Yes, of course. I believe that acupuncture and physical therapy are excellent combinations. It is part of the integrated approach that I discussed earlier.

In my clinical experience, I believe that if you have the opportunity to work with an acupuncturist, then you should decide after some visits if it helps you. Once again, it is all about the integrated and individual approach to care.

Can I continue working out?

This is different for every person, obviously. An acute back in spasm may need a day off, but exercise is paramount to the healing process. I very rarely tell my patients not to work out. You can always do something. That is where creativity comes into play. If you are working with a personal trainer, even better! Your trainer can always design a program working around your injury. Good communication is key between a physical therapist and a personal trainer.

In addition, *a good trainer knows when to refer their client to a physical therapist.* They know their skills cannot replace what a PT does. After all, it is their livelihood that will be affected if you don't show up for your session because you hurt.

What if my therapist has me coming three times a week? What if she has me continue therapy even though I feel good?

Most people's busy schedules don't even allow them to come three times a week. After all, most people are not professional athletes and do not have the need for daily physical therapy. If you feel your therapist has you coming in more than you should, then talk with your PT and find out the reason they want you to come in that many times.

However, if you are in acute back pain or you have an acute ankle sprain (you get the picture), then coming in more frequently may help. The persistent issues are the ones that I am speaking to here.

If you have had surgery, perhaps more is more, but I am of the opinion that we need to empower our patients. Encouraging thrice weekly visits not only adds to the belief that they "need" you, but it also disempowers the patient.

And that is not cool.

You are
not defined
by your
symptom

Finding the **source** vs. treating the **symptom**

Why are you treating my foot when it's my hip that hurts?
Do you mean that it is my pelvis that is causing my knee problem?

There are many barriers to the recovery process when it comes to both acute and persistent pain. One of those barriers is treating the wrong body part. You say, "What do you mean, wrong body part? My knee hurts, so shouldn't my knee be treated?" Not necessarily.

Let's say you are a golfer and your knee hurts after a long round of golf. Why does your knee hurt? Maybe you lack sufficient rotation in your mid-back in order to hit the ball through the full swing, so your low-back, hip, and knee over-rotate to compensate. In that scenario, let's say your hip is also stiff, then your knee really becomes the victim.[22]

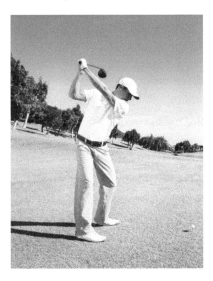

The theme throughout this book is to consider the whole person—not just the physical, but the

---

22   Marshall, Robert N. "Biomechanical risk factors and mechanisms of knee injury in golfers." Journal of Sports Biomechanics, Vol 12, Issue 3, pgs. 221-230. Feb 28, 2013.

cognitive, emotional, and social issues the person presents with. This theme or mantra ensures that we get to the source of your problem and not just treat your symptom.

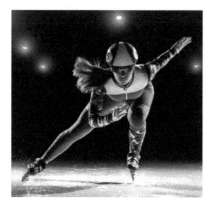

Assuming that the painful structure is the cause of your problem can lead you down the wrong path when it comes to receiving treatment. Movement is essential for many reasons, and if the painful structure is not the cause of why you cannot move well, then it behooves you to be open to an approach that will find the REAL cause of your problem.

Addressing the true source of your pain via a whole body approach contributes to more complete and lasting improvement. As you can see from the picture of this short track skater, if she has a restriction in her left hip and cannot crouch into the deep squat required by this sport, she will most likely compensate somewhere else. It would be a bit tough to do at the ankle, since she is in skates, so the body looks elsewhere to get down low. Our nervous system at its best!

Additionally, let's assume someone believes that they have to have their back cracked in order to get relief from their back pain, but they are seeing a PT for the first time and the assessment reveals that their hip is the source of their problem. That cognitive belief must be invalidated in order for the person to truly feel better while their hip is being treated and their back is not being cracked as regularly as they want.[23]

For some who have persistent pain, they think about it so much that it becomes a part of who they are, literally their identity. They self-limit their activities to the point that it really has a negative effect on their overall function. They have a strong emotional component and connection to their pain in addition to a sensitive nervous system. (More about that in the patient stories.)

---

23   Ehde, Dawn M.; Dillworth, Tiara M.; Turner, Judith A. "Cognitive-behavioral therapy for individuals with chronic pain: Efficacy, innovations, and directions for research." American Psychologist, Vol 69(2), Feb-Mar 2014, 153-166.

A sensitive nervous system must be addressed if physical therapy is to be successful for that person. As I mentioned previously in the book, pain education has come a long way in the past decade, and there are certain things that we can do as physical therapists to help overcome this particular barrier.[24]

As physiotherapists, we are trying to change the experience of how you feel in your body when you move. We are changing your strategies so that you can move and feel better. We are changing your pain experience.

If that means treating the hip or the foot for back pain or treating your thorax[25] for your knee pain, then so be it. Most of you will feel the difference when you move if the right body region has been treated.

We are looking for your "buckle point," so to speak. I am looking for a way into your nervous system. When I assess a specific movement, I look for areas of the body that are not moving optimally, moving too much, moving too little, or just not moving at all. I look at the biomechanics, control, and load/force required for that specific movement to occur. I look to see if there is strain being delivered excessively somewhere. I also look at the patient's face, as much can be gleaned from judging someone's reaction to a movement that is painful. Is it fear? Is there some other barrier that is preventing them from, for example, squatting properly?

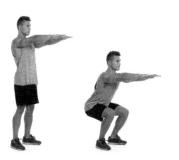

Are they afraid they are going to leak? Afraid that they will fall? That is the whole person approach—it's not just the physical.

Let's take this squat, for example. Squatting requires movement at the feet, knees, hips, pelvis, back, arms, and head.

---

24   Butler, David S. The Sensitive Nervous System. OPTP: 2006.

25   The part of the trunk between the neck and the abdomen, enclosed by the ribs, sternum, and certain vertebrae, in which the heart, lungs and other viscera are situated.

Let's say that person A has low-back pain with sitting and Person B has low-back pain while performing a squat in the gym. Same symptom, different aggravating factors. You have to get to a sitting posture via a squat, so I assess the squat for both people.

In order to compensate, Person A shifts his body weight to the right and rotates to the left to sit, and Person B also rotates to the left to get lower in the squat. Once again, this is your nervous system giving you options. Person A does this because his left side hurts when he squats (from an old rib injury). Person B does this because his left ankle is too stiff to accommodate the movement. Both have low-back pain. But what is the source of their pain? The body takes the path of least resistance, and for both of these individuals, it was their back.

Performing the assessment, looking at the whole person, and playing one area off of the other, I determine that the old rib fracture for Person A is the source and for Person B it's their ankle fracture. If I treated only their low-back pain (symptom), they would most likely not experience any long-term relief or benefit.[26]

Sometimes treating the symptomatic part may bring the patient some relief in the short-term, but that is only temporary. The pain almost always comes back. In the case of Person A and Person B, their pain would eventually return.

Treating the source of the problem not only gives you long-term relief, but it also empowers you with the knowledge and tools to help prevent your problem from returning (or not lasting long if it does return). The ultimate goal for any treatment program, no matter who you are, is to change the way you move in your body so that you can experience a full life.

" The ultimate goal for any treatment program, no matter who you are, is to change the way you move in your body so that you can experience a full life. "

---

26   Sueki, Derrick G; Cleland, Joshua A; Wainner, Robert S. "A regional interdependence model of musculoskeletal dysfunction: research, mechanisms, and clinical implications." Journal of Manual & Manipulative Therapy, Vol 21, Issue 2, 90-102: 2013.

We are trying to help you get rid of old strategies and replace them with new ones. This creates new neural networks and motor maps in your brain so that you can move with ease and grace. Consider someone who sees a physical therapist because they have a problem running. Let's say their back hurts, for example. Why would I watch them squat? Running is not squatting. The demands on the body are completely different. In the same way, why would I have them bend over to see if they can touch their toes when that has absolutely nothing to do with running?

It's all part of the process.

Whatever problem or issue that drives you to see a physical therapist, you as the patient need to understand that the PT must perform the evaluation in a way that is significant and relevant for you and them. This enables you to get the results you want and the treatment you deserve.

The premise that injury to tissues (muscle, ligament, nerve, bone, etc.) is the cause of pain gave rise to what we call the pathoanatomical model for pain.[27] Many clinicians thought that if the tissue(s) were to be treated, the pain would go away and the patient would recover. There have been significant advances in clinical neuroscience that have changed how we view pain to refute that belief. [28,29,30]

It is now recognized that this view is limited in sense and scope. A new "biopsychosocial"[31] model of pain is now more widely adapted and takes into account the whole person and not just the body part that hurts. With pain viewed as a dynamic process among and within the biological, psychological, and social factors unique to each individual, this approach gives you a much more holistic view of pain.

---

27   This model is based on pathology and focuses on the consequences of inflammation, infection, trauma disease, etc.

28   Cooper, Saths (editor); Rateie, Kopano (editor). Psychology Serving Humanity: Proceedings of the 30th International Congress of Psychology, Vol 2, Western Psychology. Psychology Press: 2014

29   Gifford, Louis. Topical Issues in Pain 3: Sympathetic Nervous System and Pain, Pain Management, Clinical Effectiveness. CNS Press: 2002.

30   Moseley, Lorimer; Butler, David. Explain Pain Supercharged. NOI Group Publications, 2017

31   Gatchel RJ, Peng YB, Peters, ML, Fuchs PN, Turk DC The Biopsychosocial Approach to Chronic Pain: Scientific Advances and Future Directions, Psychol Bull. 2007 Jul;133(4):581-624

Many people have significant back pain while their tests (X-ray, MRI, etc.) reveal nothing that could justify the amount of pain the person experiences. Remember: X-rays and MRIs do not show pain. They show you at one point in time, and you are not even moving during those tests. You are a dynamic human being. In contrast, some people who have horrific scans and X-rays walk around all day long with no pain at all. *A "chasing pain" treatment plan is simply ineffective unless it is justified by a sound clinical reasoning process.*

In some cases, our tissues heal and yet pain persists. An example of this is an ankle sprain that is still bothersome after four months. At this point, the tissues around the ankle are generally healed, yet the person still experiences pain. Moreover, treating the painful structure does not take into account other structures in the body that may be pain-free but could be the underlying cause of the problem.

Finding the source of your pain is pretty powerful; it actually tells us WHY you hurt. Isn't that what you want?

It is well-known that just because you got rid of your pain, it does not mean that you have full function. It is becoming increasing more well-known that there are many people *without pain* who want to optimize their performance. Furthermore, their performance is worth more to them than getting rid of their pain. In this instance, pain-free structures may very well be the reason why they have not achieved peak performance.

I would go so far as to say that prevention of injury and optimal performance should be the goals for everyone, whether you have pain or not. Your idea of performance could be as advanced as running a marathon or as simple as walking down the street. Performance expectations will be different for everyone. Pain is not an issue here with these people; function is the issue. That is why it is *paramount* that you ultimately get to the source of your problem.

A great example here is someone who comes into the clinic with some mild knee pain that only occurs with lunges (and it is the back leg that hurts). That is the only time that she experiences it. Stairs, running, and jumping are all fine, but she wants to compete in a trail run and just wants to make sure that this will not affect her performance. This is relevant for trails, because it is that back leg that helps propel us up.

"Performance should be the goals for everyone, whether you have pain or not."

The assessment reveals that the source to that knee pain is her hip and not the knee. The hip receives some treatment, and the patient has some tools in her toolbox to manage the mild pain in case it happens again. As it turns out, the person does the trail run and has a personal best.

Is it a coincidence? Maybe, maybe not.

I'll give you another scenario: an elite athlete, let's say a golfer, and a recreational golfer, as examples. The distinction is obvious. Both have back pain. Is the source of pain the same? It depends on the context. Let's say the original source of back pain is in the hips. They overcompensate in their back because of lack of rotation in their hips. Let's keep it simple.

The professional golfer is at the Master's, the recreational golfer is playing with friends at Torrey Pines; both are at the eighteenth hole. The pro is quieting his brain. Professional athletes know how to quiet their brains and FOCUS while the recreational golfer generally does not. Their backs are killing them, but the professional athlete knows how to dampen down their back pain. Their brain is prioritizing.

Winning the Masters is more important. The professional golfer nails the putt and wins the millions. The recreational golfer's focus is broad, and he misses the putt.

Tour players possess a unique ability to quiet their minds and control their thoughts while still being able to play at a high level.

Yes, the musculoskeletal source of their low-back pain is their hip. However, when the patient has to run the marathon, do a triathlon, compete in Olympic trials, or play in their club tournament, we must consider that there may be another source that is contributing to the problem—es*pecially if their pain is magnified during these activities.* Thoughts about pain will impact sports performance.[32]

Symptom versus source?

---

32   Smith, Mark F. Golf Science: Optimum Performance From Tee To Green. University of Chicago Press: 2013.

Both the professional golfer and the recreational golfer had the same symptom (low-back pain) and the same source (hip). That may be all it takes to get them back on the course pain-free. The recreational golfer, however, still gets his back pain when he plays. The professional golfer does not. At this point, the answer lies in how he is processing the pain while on the golf course, not in treating his low-back. The hip looks good, and there seem to be no other physical sources of the back pain, so what happens on the golf course or at the eighteenth hole with the recreational golfer?

This is where you need to consider an *additional source* to the problem—the power of the brain and its relationship to pain. The brain weighs in on whether or not the current situation is dangerous enough for the individual to cause them pain. It is akin to spraining your ankle and then seeing a bear. You are more concerned with running away from the bear than you are with the ankle. Make sense?[33,34]

I don't want to get too technical here with this concept as it is beyond the scope of the book. However, the professional golfer's brain is more concerned with winning the tournament. It prioritizes. That is something you must train. Focus, discipline, and brain training are all a part of rehab.

We need to train motor control and place the patient in the context within which they experience pain, either literally or simulated. That way they can retrain their brain and develop a new motor map. The distinction is how to focus and quiet their brain.[35]

Put the professional golfer on the Wii or in a simulated tournament and train that brain to focus and mitigate the distractions. Do the same thing with the recreational golfer, a cyclist, a tennis player—any form of athlete. With this type of training over time, he will learn how to focus and down-regulate his nervous system to take the focus off his back and put the focus on the putt when he plays, cycles up that tough hill, or hits the

---

33   Mosely, G. Lorimer; Butler, David S. The Journal Of Pain - Fifteen Years of Explaining Pain, Vol 16, Issue 9, 807-813. 2015.

34   Asmundson, Gordon (editor); Viaeyen, Johan (editor); Cronbez, Geert (editor). Understanding and Treating Fear of Pain: Role of Hypervigilance and Fear of Pain, 1st edition. Oxford University Press: 2004.

35   Testa, Marco; Rossettini, Giacomo. "Enhance placebo, avoid nocebo: How contextual factors affect physiotherapy outcomes." Manual Therapy, Vol 24, 65-74. Elsevier, Ltd: 2016.

winning backhand. That will decrease his back pain and increase sports performance, for sure.[36,37]

When someone is in chronic pain, they develop a certain set of beliefs, true or not, that ultimately slow down their healing. There is a saying, "If you are in pain, and you live your pain with constant focus, you get more pain." The fear of pain is worse than the pain itself.[38]

If you think that the source of your back pain is your back and the physical assessment reveals that it is not, please be open to the possibility that there are other sources to your problem, even if it means training your brain out of pain.

Keep in mind that we are learning to consider the whole person, not just the symptomatic area. The painful structure may not be the cause of the problem. In the following patient stories, we will discuss not just the physical, but the cognitive, emotional, and social issues the person presents with. Rather than just treating the symptom, we get to the source of the problem with a whole body approach that is more likely to lead to complete and lasting improvement.

And isn't that what you want? Is that not your priority?

If you find yourself wondering why your symptoms and/or your performance is not improving, whether it is sports related or not, then read on. You will discover the value of treating the source of your problem rather than just your symptom.

---

36   http://www.bodyinmind.org/wp-content/uploads/The-Australian_The-champion-cyclist.pdf

37   Ericsson, KA Training history, deliberate practice and elite sports performance: an analysis in response to Tucker and Collins review—what makes champions? *Br J Sports Med*, 47, 533-535;July 14, 2014.

38   Crombez, Geert; Eccleston, Christopher; Van Damme, Stefaan; Viaeyen, Yohan; Karoly, Paul. "Fear Avoidance Model of Chronic Pain: The Next Generation." Clinical Journal of Pain, Vol 28, Issue 6, 475-483. Lippincott Wiliams & Wilkins: 2012.

Healing
comes from
within

Chapter 1

Really? My **neck** pain is coming from my **shoulder blade**?

Neck pain does not always originate in the neck. It can come from other parts of your upper body or start with a compensation[39] from your low-back or rib cage, for example.

Truth

Neck pain and its associated restrictions can literally be a *pain in the neck*! But in some cases—such as neck pain that comes and goes, or neck pain that won't go away despite treatment to the neck—the source may lie elsewhere. Such was the situation with this person's story.

Can you see from this picture that even the slightest change in one part of the body can certainly impact another? Or try it yourself; stand with your legs straight and then bend one knee. Feel what happens to the rest of your body.

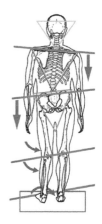

When you look down to read or turn your head to one side, movement occurs at the joints in your neck, as well as your collarbones, your upper rib cage, your shoulder joint, your shoulder blade, and even your head.

---

39   A compensation occurs when a muscle or joint is unable to perform through a specific range of motion. The body then tries to use other parts of the kinetic chain to perform whatever task or function that is necessary.

What if the source of your inability to turn your head is due to your collarbone (or clavicle) not moving as the result of an old injury sustained years ago? For example, perhaps you fell off a horse resulting in a fracture to the collarbone. And now, for some reason, when you look down or turn your head, you notice that performing this repetitive movement over and over is now restricted. Suddenly what is preventing your recovery is that old issue that has cropped up.

You say, "Well that was years ago, why would that affect me now?"

Good question. Yes, the body does adapt very well; however, changes in our daily routine can trigger old injuries. As we become involved in new activities, start a job that is either more physical or more sedentary than before, or just because we get older, we find that we cannot compensate for these injuries as well as before.

" Changes in our daily routine can trigger old injuries. "

The source of your restricted neck movement could also be due to some tight muscles attached to your shoulder blade, for example, or an eyeglass prescription that's wearing out. What do eyeglasses have to do with neck movement restrictions? When you are constantly straining to see, you tend to peer forward, altering the mechanics in the neck.

Does that necessarily cause pain? No, it doesn't. It depends on you— your genetics, your makeup, your brain, and your ability to control your reaction to pain. Some people may get a headache, others won't. Each individual processes pain differently. As a matter of fact, studies show that how you process pain will have a significant impact on your outcomes.[40,41]

As I brought up earlier in the book, twists are everywhere in our body. And this is much more evident when it comes to the neck, because our

---

40   Roussel, Nathalie A.; Nijs, Jo; Meeus, Mira; Mylius, Veit; Fayt, Cecile; Oostendorp, Rob. "Central Sensitization and Altered Central Pain Processing in Chronic Low-Back Pain: Fact or Myth?" Clinical Journal of Pain, Vol 29, Issue 7, -625-638. July 2013.

41   Carroll, Linda; Ferrari, Robert; Cassidy, J. David; Cote, Pierre. "Coping and Recovery in Whiplash-associated Disorders: Early Use of Passive Coping Strategies is Associated with Slower Recovery of Neck Pain and Pain-related Disability." Clinical Journal of Pain, Volume 30, Issue 1, 1-8. Jan 2014.

head and neck are our "crown," so to speak.

Our bodies are so good at compensating for restricted movement that sometimes we feel like we are chasing our own tail—literally. Remember: don't chase pain—it's not a good path to follow.

So what's the takeaway here?

An evaluation of someone with neck complaints is not COMPLETE unless the practitioner looks at these other areas as well.

Story

I recently had a patient who came in complaining of numbness in her fingers and shooting pain down her arm to the pinky on her left side. She also had an uncomfortable feeling on the left side of her neck and upper shoulder. She had been in PT somewhere else for almost a year and was minimally improving. She was a college student who played softball.

The patient was unable to look down to read or even to use her smartphone without pain going down her arm. She also was unable to turn her head to the left without feeling "something weird," as she put it.

An MRI was performed, which revealed a herniated disc in her neck.

Remember: treat the PERSON, not the piece of paper. Images are points in time and YOU, the person, are dynamic and moving.

There are many people who walk around all day long with lousy necks and function fine. Conversely, I have patients who are in extreme pain, yet their imaging is pristine. A person's story and their symptoms are more important than any result of imaging. If you get too hung up on what you see on an MRI or an X-ray, it could potentially slow down your recovery.

> "Images are points in time and YOU, the person, are dynamic and moving."

This patient was pretty resilient and extremely compliant with therapy. She educated the trainers on her softball team as to the cause of the problem so that they could help her during training sessions as well as pre- and post-game.

What I Found

In the type of evaluation that I perform, I ask the patient to share the one thing they cannot do that they would like to be able to do. It's not a difficult question per se. With some patients there are many answers to this question, so we prioritize.

In this instance, the patient answered, "I cannot look down or turn my head to the left." These are two different tasks with many different physical requirements.

When I performed the evaluation on this patient, certain restrictions and weaknesses appeared. Since the movements that were most significant for her were looking down and turning her head to the left, those were the motions I evaluated.

When you look down to read or work on your laptop computer, movement has to occur at many joints. During an evaluation, I am looking for the buckle point or the most vulnerable point, so to speak. Our bodies are great compensators and often take the path of least resistance until we can't compensate anymore. Our brains are really smart that way. We find different options for movement and our nervous systems adjust.

The findings that were most relevant to determining the cause of her inability to look down or turn her head to the left were the following.

She had some restrictions in her upper thorax (the area of the body between the neck and lower back), which were limiting her ability to look down as well as turn to the left. To possibly compensate for this, as the brain often does, it sought to get the mobility elsewhere. Sometimes we try and turn our entire shoulder complex to the left or we bring our left shoulder blade back to sneak out that extra bit of movement, which was the case with her. Once again, the beauty of our nervous system.

These findings mean nothing to the average person. All they know is that they can't do what they want to do because it hurts. They feel "off."

When dealing with this kind of pain, one might think, *This is not so bad, I can compensate for all this.* Or perhaps it happens at a deeper level in the brain, with the body following directions as to how it can compensate to avoid the pain.

In the case of this patient, she was a softball player who functions in more than a 3-D plane. She had to coordinate multiple joints in an effort to swing the bat (turn head to the left) or look down to field a ground ball.

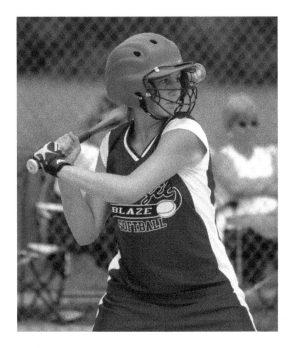

To determine which of the above findings made any sense to treat, I had to find the source(s) of the problem. I played one finding off the other, making modifications to her movement in order for her to feel better and make the movement more ideal.

Ultimately, what we found was that the primary source of her problem did lie in the compensations she made with her shoulder blade and secondarily her thorax (see page 29 for definition).

What Worked

In order to get her functional and pain-free, we had to treat the primary source—her shoulder blade—and then treat the secondary source of pain: the first through third ribs on her left side (part of her thorax). The ultimate goal of any treatment program is to adopt a new, more optimal strategy for movement. In order to do that, any obstacles that are preventing the patient from learning a new exercise or adapting to a new way of moving must be removed.

> " The ultimate goal of any treatment program is to adopt a new, more optimal strategy for movement. "

What I did

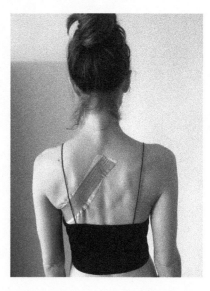

- Tape to take the load off the shoulder blade so the muscles around the area could work more effectively[42]

- Soft tissue releases to the muscles in the area, as they were holding the shoulder blade in a non-optimal position

- Mobility techniques to the restricted areas in and around the shoulder girdle, in an effort to increase movement and allow the muscles, nerves, and joints to move effectively

- Soft tissue release to muscles such as the serratus anterior and pectoralis minor (see next page), as they were restricting her ability to turn her head to the left.

---

42   Lee, Diane and Lee, Linda Joy (LJ). *Discover Physio Series*, Vancouver, B.C., 2012.

Training requires repetition to make it habitual, so to speak.[43] Not only does repetitive movement reinforce a good movement pattern for the patient, but after a while it becomes the norm and is performed subconsciously. Above all, the movement has to be appropriate for the patient in the sense that it is relevant to the activity that she cannot perform currently without pain.

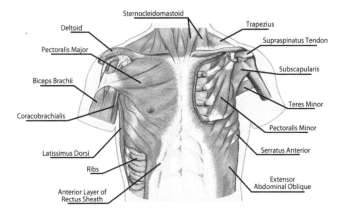

" Keep in mind: Using the brain in training is über important! Mindless work here will not get results. "

In the case of my patient, she could not look down, so we devised easier starting points for her exercise program—lying on her back, on her hands and knees. I trained her on some unloaded exercises and we progressed her from there.

Keep in mind: Using the brain in training is über important! Mindless work here will not get results.

---

43   Bayona, Nestor A.; Bitensky, Jamie; Salter, Katherine; Teasell, Robert. "The Role of Task-Specific Training in Rehabilitation Therapies." Topics in Stroke Rehab, Vol 12, Issue3: 2005.

A sample of some of the corrective exercises for this particular patient could include (note: these are relevant for her):

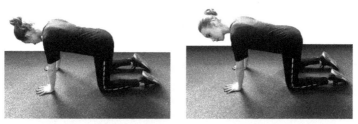

Getting on all fours and slowly dropping the head down and also turning to the left

This achieves the goal of movement and gets her head to move better in a different context[44,45] than she is used to. While she is dropping her head, she cues herself to "soften (relax) her shoulder blade." She can also turn her head to the left side in this position.

You want to use the words that make sense for you. In this case, when she thought of softening the shoulder blade, she was able to look down with increased pain-free motion.

Again, it is very important to be mindful during each movement as this engages the brain and will ultimately build a better motor pattern.

One could also do a Modified Down Dog and slowly drop the head down. This movement has the added benefit of training control of her secondary issue, her thorax. Putting our hands down like this, in a supported position on the floor, helps elongate and soften the rib cage.

The downward dog movement can be made more difficult through progression by performing it on a Pilates Reformer and then moving onto one leg, increasing the load. Even harder!

44   Carlino, E.; Benedetti, F. "Different contexts, different pains, different experiences." Neuroscience. Elsevier, Ltd.: Dec 2016.

45   Davids, Keith; Araujo, Duarte; Correia, Vanda; Villar, Luis. "How Small-Sided and Conditioned Games Enhance Acquistion of Movement and Decision-Making Skills." Exercise and Sport Science Reviews, Vol 41, Issue 3, 154-161. July 2013.

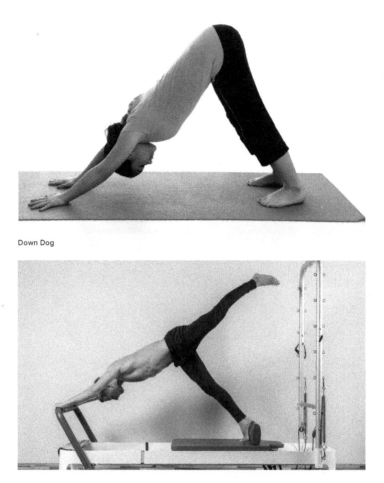

Down Dog

In order to open up her upper chest, we added a triangle pose to the left. You can see from the picture on the next page that this movement really elongates the torso which, in turn, helps facilitate the neck rotation to the left that she desired. It is also a great way to incorporate a new movement pattern and train the brain. If you remember from the chapter "Finding the Source vs. Treating the Symptom," training your brain is vital because it helps you get rid of old strategies and replace them with new ones, creating new neural networks and motor maps in your brain, so that you can move with ease and grace. And that's something we all want!

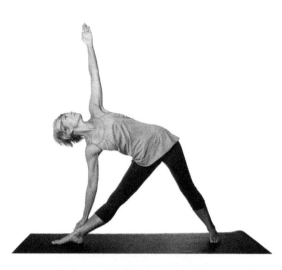

Positive Results

- Ability to use her Smartphone without symptoms

- Ability to look down and field ground balls without pain.

- Ability to turn her head to the left without problems; this helped her softball ability as well!

- Understanding of what to do to not only *prevent* this from happening again but also *what she could do to manage it* if it did

Pain is a
**public health
concern**

Chapter 2

Really? My **neck** hurts because of a tight **pectoral muscle**?

Did you know that your neck pain and perhaps your inability to turn your head (while driving) could be caused by tightness in the muscles of your chest?

Truth

As I mentioned in the previous story, neck pain may not originate in your neck. Often it does; sometimes it does not. When you have neck pain that is persistent, the issue is generally multifaceted and there are likely other contributors to your problem. Please be open to this possibility.

One of these contributors could be tightness or restriction in the muscles and joints of your upper chest or upper neck. Another factor could be

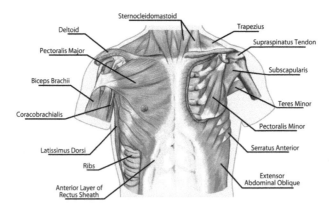

a restriction in the mobility of your collarbones (clavicles) from an old fracture there, tightness in the pectoral muscles in your chest from doing too many bench presses at the gym, or just from simple daily activities.

If you think about it, most of the activities we experience as a part of daily living are in the front of our bodies: writing, computer work, sitting at our desks, talking on our phones. As you can see from the picture on the preceding page, these muscles are closely connected to your neck. That is why it is crucial to acknowledge the influence these muscles have on your neck and its ability to move. To ignore the effect that these muscles have on your neck movement would be incomplete, not to mention the effect it has on our spatial representation in our brains. If we spend our day performing tasks in front of our body, our brain thinks this is normal. When we change the position or context of movement, like turning our heads to look for a passing car, for example, our brains register this as "new" or "novel."

That's not to say that these restrictions are causing your pain, but you need to consider the kinetic chain and how one body part affects the other, and this includes the brain. Certain postural positions tend to place our center of mass forward and our body schema—a representation of our body parts in space—generally changes.

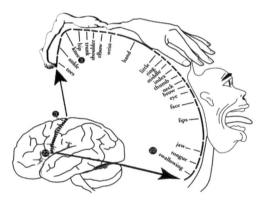

Homonculus, original work from Dr. Wilder Penfield

Simply put, a body schema can be considered the collection of brain processes that registers the position of one's body parts in space. The schema is updated during body movement. This is typically a nonconscious process, and is used primarily for spatial organization of action.[46,47]

In general, and in the examples above—sitting at a desk, writing, etc.—our center of mass is forward. When we actually do something that takes us out of our "normal" forward position, we find it "weird" or "off." Unless we do activities to counteract or counterbalance these postures, we will tend to have an overall pull forward.

Another example is when we compensate and put more weight on one leg because of an injury; after we rehab it and equalize our weight bearing, it may feel strange because it is something we are not used to. That just takes training and time before it becomes our new normal.

Our tendency is to "jut" our heads forward to see the screen, phone, etc. What this does, in effect, is tighten (shorten) the muscles in our upper neck.

Here is a nice example of a counterbalancing posture:

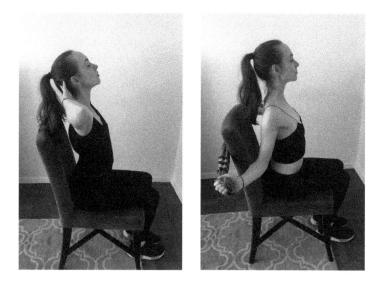

46   Wallwork, Sarah B.; Bellan, Valeria; Catley, Mark J.; Mosely, G. Lorimer. Neural representations and the cortical body matrix: implications for sports medicine and future directions." British Journal of Sports Medicine, Dec 2015.

47   Morasso, Paetro; Casadio, Maura; Mohan, Vishwanathan; Rea, Francesco; Zenzeri, Jacopo. "Revisiting the Body-Schema Concept in the Context of the Whole-Body Postural-Focal Dynamics." Frontiers in Human Neuroscience, 2015.

To give you a real-life example, let's consider the daily activity of backing out of your driveway or a parking space. When you turn your head to the left and over your shoulder to check for cars or other obstructions, you are tensioning—opening and/or stretching—the front of your chest and the right side of your neck. If there is a movement restriction present, then you will compensate in order to make sure there are no cars in your way. Your brain figures out a way to get that done.

"Persistent thoughts about pain will change our brain maps. "

Over time, compensations occur and because of this, you may have discomfort on the left side of your neck because you are trying to force the movement. But the real cause can be on your opposite side. If this pain has been persistent, which means it has lasted for months, you may have developed physical compensations as well as a belief that it will never get better.

Just know, it will get better.

Persistent thoughts about pain will change our brain maps. Have you ever noticed that when you get distracted you don't necessarily feel your pain?[48] Your thoughts are diverted. Intensely focusing on pain will not make us better. In fact, it will set us back. This is a whole other topic (and another book!), but just know that if we are in control of our thoughts about our pain, we are on the way to recovery.

Story

A patient of mine complained that she could not turn her head to the left. Just as in the example above, she experienced this pain when she was backing her car up or changing lanes on a highway. In addition, her job was more sedentary, and she tended to turn to the right while she was working at her computer. While at the office, she had a generally forward and right-sided bias. This right-side bias continued at home when she watched TV, due to the location of the television.

---

48   Sprenger, Christian; Eppert, Falk; Finsterbusch, Jurgen; Bingel, Ulrike; Rose, Michael; Buchel, Christian. "Pain Relief Through Distraction: It's not all in your head." Current Biology, 2012.

Over the years she had chronic neck pain, which resolved on its own. However, since she had changed jobs, the pain was not resolving as usual.

Common sense would dictate I ask, "What is she doing differently that she has not done before? Could it be her office setup?" Apparently, the ergonomics of her office had changed, and she found herself turning more to the right because of her phone and computer location.

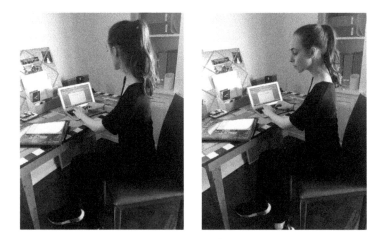

Sometimes we don't realize that what we do all day is a contributing factor to our symptoms. Our habits and movement patterns over time are important. In her case, it was one of the major causes of her restriction.

Note in the photo above, that if you constantly turn your body to the right all day because of your work positioning, you will develop a bias towards that side. Although her chair is positioned to the left, her upper body has rotated to the right; with her left leg crossed over the right, this position becomes even more reinforced.

Please note that not all people who sit this way have pain, and everyone is different. All people sit differently. Just because someone sits one way, that does not mean they will have pain. As a physiotherapist, I decide if it is relevant based on their story and symptoms.

Over time, your joints and muscles will adapt. This adaptation will surface when all of a sudden you have to do a task that requires rotation to the left on a consistent basis. In the patient's case, the adaptation surfaced when she had to turn her head to the left to back out of her driveway or change lanes on a highway.

In her prior job, she did not have these non-optimal ergonomics, and thus was able to compensate when she had to drive her car. It's easy to compensate because our brains handle it flawlessly without us even knowing.

What I Found

The initial evaluation revealed significant tightness in the muscles of her chest (pectorals), and a tendency to sit or stand with her upper body turned slightly to the right. No big deal—that is common. That is how she spent most of the day at her desk. When her movement was assessed, it seemed that this bias predominated throughout.

The motion that I assessed was turning her head to the left—or in my lingo, rotation left. It is important to assess the motion or movement that is relevant for you, the patient. It validates why you came in. Right? It would not make sense if I had assessed, for example, looking down as if reading a book, as in the other neck story. That movement was actually pain-free for her and would not be useful information in this case.

When you turn your head to the left, movement occurs at many joints. Not only does your neck turn left, but your head and shoulder girdle turn as well. The collarbones (or clavicles) will also move when one is turning the head. It is not a lot of movement, but there is a certain amount of rotation that should occur. If there is a restriction somewhere, our brains try and get the rotation elsewhere (i.e., the neck or the upper ribs). That is our nervous system at its best. It finds another way for us to move. This can cause compensatory problems and a breakdown in the kinetic chain may occur.

> But let's be clear. There are people who do this all day long and have no neck pain at all.

In the following picture, look at how much compression could possibly occur in the upper neck and anterior chest if one sits like this for a prolonged period of time and over many years! Just to keep the eyes looking straight ahead at your computer, you would to have to move your neck in ways that could potentially be non-optimal. Imagine doing that year after year.

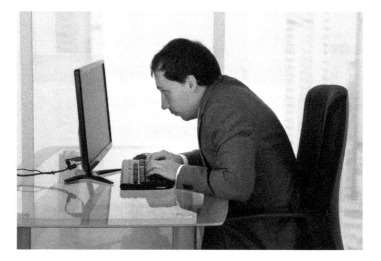

But let's be clear. There are people who do this all day long and have no neck pain at all. It is important to remember that we are all heterogeneous individuals and what works for someone else may not work for you. Personally, if I sit like that all day, my neck and shoulders hurt and I have a headache. You may sit like that and be perfectly fine. It all goes back to the concept of strategy. We find different strategies so that we can sit and feel better. Our nervous system is constantly adjusting.

We all have different buckle points, and that is what makes us unique. The key to good posture, whether it is sitting or standing, is to vary or change your position often. There is no right way to sit or stand. The key is to mix it up.

It is the responsibility of the physical therapist to assess and find that buckle point and to treat it accordingly. If you are being treated for neck pain and have not fully recovered, then please ask your therapist to look elsewhere for the source(s) of your problem.

For this patient, the following findings were most relevant after my assessment:

- Muscle and joint restrictions in her upper body that were limiting her ability to turn her head to the left (clavicles, sternocleidomastoid, and upper trapezius muscles: see photo on page 48).

- Additionally, soft tissue restrictions included tightness in the pectoral (chest) muscles, and other muscles in the upper chest that were also impeding her ability to turn her head to the left.

- There was also some limited mobility in the joints and muscles of her upper neck (in my lingo, cranio-vertebral joints).

- Clearly, her office environment was a factor and needed to be addressed.

I modified each area of restriction above and noticed how that affected her movement to the left as well as her subjective sensation of pain. Once the assessment was finished, I determined that the upper part of her rib cage and chest was the primary source of her problem and, secondarily, her upper neck.

What Worked

My plan began with addressing the primary source of her problem, the upper rib cage and chest, as determined by my assessment. Again, the ultimate goal of any treatment program is to adopt a new, more optimal strategy for movement while correcting and addressing each area of concern. It is all about changing how you move and giving your brain new and novel options for movement.

What I did

- Soft tissue release to the muscles in the anterior (pec minor, intercostals) and lateral chest—releasing these muscles enabled her to free up some movement so she could turn her head better

- Mobilization techniques[49] to free up any remaining joint restrictions, especially in her upper neck.

- Taping of the upper rib cage to support the release and mobility work that was done.[50] Remember that the ribs are at the front and back of your body.

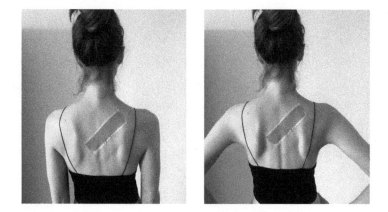

---

49   Joint mobilization is a manual therapy intervention, a type of passive movement of a skeletal joint. It is usually aimed at a 'target' synovial joint with the aim of achieving a therapeutic effect. When applied to the spine, it is known as spinal mobilization. https://en.wikipedia.org/wiki/Joint_mobilization

50   Lee, Diane and Lee, Linda Joy (LJ). *Discover Physio Series*, Vancouver, B.C., 2012.

- Prescription of corrective exercise, which included postural control and control into left rotation

Depending on the severity of the symptoms, we could have started with head and neck rotation in a different context, such as turning the head to the left while on hands and knees.

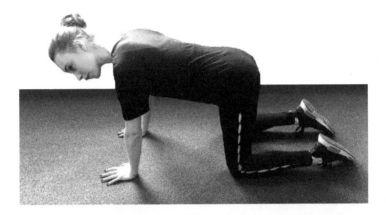

Performing a painful movement like this out of context, versus when one is sitting, helps train the brain to increase movement.[51] It's a similar motion, but it is not the one typically used when backing out of the driveway, in the case of my patient. Training rotation in this type of movement pattern helps the brain build new motor maps and ultimately helps you get better quicker.

Another option would be lower trunk rotation with your head turning to the opposite side, almost like wringing out a towel.

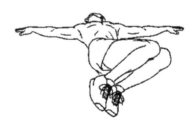

While performing these movements, it is important to connect with the source of her problem. In her case, I had her visualize more

---

51   Carlino, E.; Benedetti, F. "Different contexts, different pains, different experiences." Neuroscience. Elsevier, Ltd.: Dec 2016.

space in her upper ribs. This is the cue that worked for her; it could be different for you.

Put simply, this can be called neuromuscular reeducation or brain training. Connecting the movement with visualization techniques is very powerful and really helps solidify the new movement pattern. This kind of mindful work must be done or it just won't stick.

My secondary treatment plan included a much-needed modification to her office setup to decrease and/or eliminate the poor ergonomics. She moved some things around on her desk so as to minimize the constant shift to the right. A little goes a long way here!

Positive Results

- She can now turn her head while driving!

- She feels "more aligned" at work and during her yoga classes.

- She is able to perform certain yoga postures easier and better now that she is more aware of her bias, so to speak.

To achieve **full health** treat the **whole person**

Chapter 3

Really? My **low-back** pain is coming from my **neck**?

Would you be surprised if I told you that your lower back pain could be caused by a problem in your neck?

Truth

I put this patient in the book because her story is one that really shows the beauty of the kinetic chain and the brain. How could someone's back pain be caused by the neck?

Pain is tricky, and it doesn't always come from the place you think it does!

I would treat your neck if I felt it relevant to your back pain, and in this case, I did. This person's primary source of back pain was her neck, and she had some secondary issues, as you will see.

You can see from the picture at right that this squat is all wrong for many reasons. Notice the head position: would you squat with your head so far forward like that? I doubt you would, unless you decided to watch TV while you squatted. And that's all wrong for other reasons.

The reason I put this picture of a squat in is that my patient had back pain that became worse with sitting. You have to squat in order to sit down. If you sit down over and over again like this, your brain thinks this is normal.

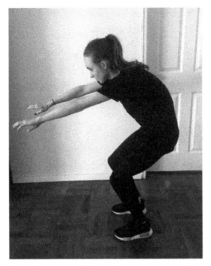

As I have mentioned in the other parts of this book, the body and brain adapt. These adaptations are what cause the persistent issues you have that eventually lead you to seek out a physical therapist. Remember: *Physical therapists are the experts in movement.* The spine does not exist in isolation; there are many forces that act upon it, including the neck.

When we sit, we generally are doing something while we sit. These days most people are looking down at their phones, at work on a computer, or reading, etc. They are not just sitting and doing nothing. What a novelty! Some quiet time. As a side note, I put forth that if we had more quiet meditative time in our lives we would have less pain.

As mentioned previously, it is estimated that the economic cost of persistent pain in the United States is between $560 and $635 billion dollars![52] The patient in this story certainly saw many practitioners in her quest for some answers and most likely paid out of pocket for a majority of that care.

Our bodies have interconnecting systems (brain, joints, viscera, etc.), and these systems are the ones that provide a link from one body part to the other. All of these links work together to provide our body with stability and/or mobility depending on the demands of each task. That is our nervous system hard at work, trying to maximize our movement potential with the appropriate amount of effort from our body.

---

52   Gaskin, Darrell J.; Richard, Patrick. "The Economic Costs of Pain in the United States." Journal of Pain, Vol 13, Issue 8, 715-724. August 2012.

" As a side note, I put forth that if we had more quiet meditative time in our lives we would have less pain. "

If we have an adaptation in our neck, for example, due to constantly turning to one side at our desks or from past trauma, our low-back is just one area that will compensate to adjust for this movement pattern.

They say that we are only as strong as our weakest link. The low-back or lumbar spine is, in my experience, an area that is often the victim. The body takes the path of least resistance and oftentimes with chronic spinal issues, it is the low-back that is the weak link.[53]

Taking a Band-Aid approach by just treating the symptoms with issues such as these will not work. They did not work for my patient, as she had seen multiple MDs, chiropractors, and physical therapists in her quest for relief.

Story

This patient came to me over a year ago with chronic right-sided low-back pain—and I mean CHRONIC. She had it for years. Can you imagine? She had made the obligatory rounds to other health care practitioners, including her OB/GYN and gastroenterologist, without much relief or explanation of her symptoms.

Her past medical history consisted of an abdominal infection as well as laparoscopic surgery. As directed, she had been performing traditional pelvic floor exercises, which she felt were making her condition worse. Seemingly, no one was able to help her. She admitted that she was at her wits' end.

" Providing pain education can be de-threatening and will help progress treatment and help with compliance. "

She was unable to sit for long periods—though she sat for most of the day at work—or walk long distances. As walking was her main form of

---

53   Sahrmann, Shirley, *Diagnosis and Treatment of Movement Impairment Syndromes*, Elsevier Health Services: 2001, p. 51.

exercise, this was depressing and discouraging for her. In addition, she was unable to bend forward or sit in her car without feeling a nagging sense of pain on her right side.

Clearly, when patients have this type of scenario—persistent pain and a feeling that no one can help them—there are other factors influencing their rate of recovery. Fear of movement and doing anything that will worsen their pain is high on their list. A persistent pain scenario such as this one is often accompanied by the influence of psychological and social variables.[54]

Providing pain education can be de-threatening and will help progress treatment and help with compliance. Knowledge is power and really helped in this case.

What I Found

When I performed the initial assessment, I found a restriction in the patient's head and neck that was contributing to her problem. When she went through a series of assessments that were similar to sitting and walking, the area that was most dysfunctional was her neck. I played one area off of other areas; when her head/neck position was modified, her pain diminished and the movements felt more fluid to her.

Most relevant findings:

- Muscular restrictions in her hip and abdomen (Remember, she had prior laparoscopic surgery?)

- Restrictions in some of her upper neck muscles (suboccipital in PT language) as well as her lower neck muscles

- Joint restrictions in her neck

- Poor movement or control in her low-back when she bent forward and when she squatted

With the use of a mirror, she was able to see this impaired movement, which was most evident during a squat. The minute she started to sit, her

---

54   O'Sullivan, Peter; Lin, Ivan. "Acute low-back pain: Beyond drug therapies." Pain Management Today, Vol 1, No 1, 2014.

neck shifted to the right. When the body senses this disequilibrium, it tries to rectify it by increasing or decreasing movement and/or control in another area. In her case, that other area was her lower back.

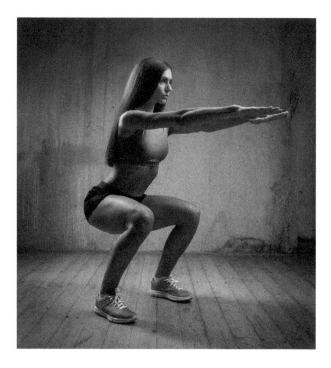

See how this is similar to the sitting posture?

When I modified her neck in the squat, she felt lighter and better in her body. We also made adjustments to the way that she walked. Prior to correcting her walking habit, she would frequently look downwards while walking, and this caused back pain. This resulted in a pull from her neck down to her back and was most likely caused by a prior foot problem that made her more aware of her foot while she walked. Remember the significance of a prior injury?

In this case, the primary cause of her low-back issue was her neck and, secondarily, the restrictions in her abdomen. It is important to note the soft tissue restrictions in her abdomen. One cannot underestimate the pull of scar tissue, especially in this case, as it was to a lesser extent a contributing factor in her low-back pain.

What Worked

I started this person's program by addressing the primary issue first, her neck. This was done via a combination of manual therapy techniques to the muscles and joints of her neck as well as specific nerve glides[55] relevant to sitting (Nerve glides are specifically designed movement techniques that restore the mobility of peripheral nerves.) Although she did not have a nerve injury per se, I believe that we need to keep our nervous system happy.

She also had a home program that included a progression of the nerve glides as well as a squat progression with some visualization techniques to help her alleviate her back pain with sitting. Progression of her corrective exercise program included weight shifting onto her left leg and then eventually some single-leg balance to help with the walking task.

What I did

- Nerve glides (see photo below) and manual therapy to the muscles and joints of the neck

- Squat progression that included a cue to take away back pain while sitting

- Progression of corrective exercise, which included weight shifting onto left leg and eventually single-leg balance to help with walking

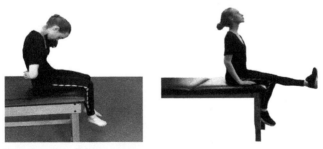

Nerve glides-Slump Sliders

---

55   Butler, David S. *The Sensitive Nervous System*, NOI Group Publications: 2000, Adelaide.

Additionally, we could have done some leg presses on the Pilates reformer with the head in neutral. It is important to note that these movements should be done in a mindful manner with focus on form. *Practice makes permanent.*

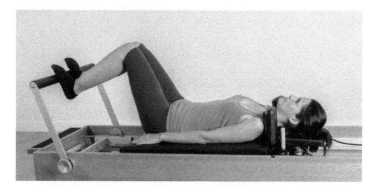

This positioning simulates the squat in an unloaded, supported, and less threatening posture. Changing up the exercise program in this way is important for the brain. It creates new motor maps, and that helps a patient to heal and recover more quickly.

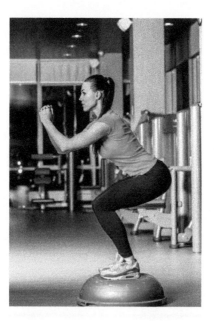

Or see photo on previous page for another way to progress the squat to a more challenging surface. And even better on a BOSU ball! Furthermore, squatting and then going to a wider stance on a moving Pilates reformer is indeed difficult. This trains the weight shift I mentioned above. (See photo below.)

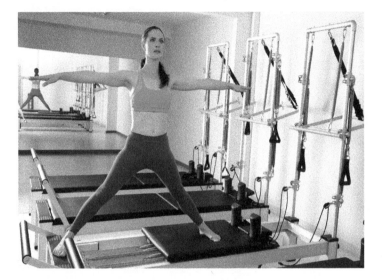

We could have also done some Pilates roll downs on the Cadillac to work on her sitting posture and neck flexibility.

Pain Education

I am a firm believer in educating my patients about pain. Why do they have it? Why has it persisted so long, and why won't it go away?

As I mentioned before, knowledge about your pain can help de-threaten movement, give you an increased sense of control, and reduce your sense of fear surrounding certain movements that you won't do because you think it will hurt.[56]

Everyone's situation is unique and their response to pain varies widely. In her case we discussed certain reasons why her pain had persisted so

---

56   Butler, David; Moseley, Lorimer. *Explain Pain*. NOI Group: 2013.

long and the distress she felt after seeing so many practitioners without any long-term relief. I believe that with her, reassurance that she would get better and the knowledge that her pain did not equal harm was a contributing factor in her recovery.

Additional Treatment

Since I believed that her abdominal surgery was a secondary issue, I included soft tissue work to her abdomen to release some of the scar tissue. She told me that this helped quite a bit. The triangle pose in yoga would also help her recovery, as it would help open up and elongate the sides of her lower rib cage where the scarring was.

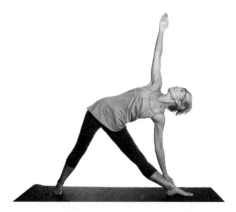

Doing different forms of breath work helped her as well. We did some diaphragmatic breathing, but you could do other types as well. It has been shown that breathing relaxes the nervous system,[57] which in turn can help dampen down some of the tone in her abdomen and the pelvic floor, which was one of our goals.

---

57   Busch, V., Magerl, W., Kern, U., Haas, J., Hajak, G. and Eichhammer, P. "The Effect of Deep and Slow Breathing on Pain Perception, Autonomic Activity, and Mood Processing—An Experimental Study." Pain Medicine, 13: 215–228. doi:10.1111/j.1526-4637.2011.01243.x. (2012).

Positive Results

- The ability to sit and walk for longer periods of time

- A new set of tools to use in case the pain returns

- A feeling of being *empowered* and *educated*

- *Best of all ... to quote my client: "I have my life back!"*

Focused practice makes **permanent,** not **perfect**

Chapter 4

Really? My **back** hurts because of a tight **hip** and **foot**?

Did you know that if you experience low-back pain while you play golf or tennis, it could be coming from a dysfunction in your foot or somewhere higher up?

Truth

At this point in the book, I think you realize that I am a big proponent of looking up and down the proverbial chain for the answer to your pain problem. You may think, *The hip and foot causing my low-back pain in golf ... and tennis? Really?* Yes, really.

The foot has to move in the golf swing—maybe not so much in putting, but definitely through the swing. The same goes for tennis, if not more! Anyone who plays golf will appreciate the movement that has to occur at the top of the backswing into the follow-through. Both feet have to move. Different movements, to be sure, but movement none the less.

Although they have the same moving parts, tennis is different from golf in its speed, force, and control of the ball.

As you can see from both pictures on the next page, a great deal of rotation is involved with these sports, from the foot all the way up to the head. Superimpose that rotation on a narrow to a wide base of support, and you have different forces going through your system.

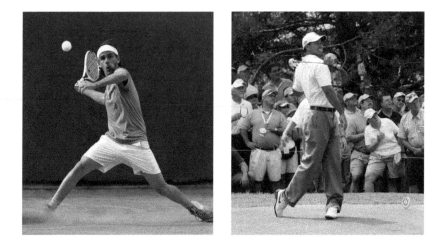

These repetitive swing patterns can predispose a golfer, or anyone participating in a rotary sport, to considerable spinal load, and players with a history of low-back pain tend to have different swing mechanics than those without.[58]

Our back and our hips often tend to get stressed more than usual. If you have a joint or muscle dysfunction somewhere in your body, but it is pain-free, it can still affect other parts of your system. This is especially true if you do the same repeated movements over and over again.

For example, you fractured your ankle years ago; it is now healed and pain-free. Yet you still feel it stiffen up every so often. You start a new exercise program where you are squatting and/or deadlifting. After a while, your back starts to bother you because your foot is so stiff, you can't get to the bottom of your squat, so you weight shift to the other side to complete the motion. Do that often enough, and something has to give—if you can't control it.

As I have stated before in the other stories, the body takes the path of least resistance. If you continue in the same vein for years, you will develop a susceptibility to a certain movement pattern. Anyone who plays golf or tennis can attest to this. If you take a moment to check your rotation dur-

58   Yung-Shen, Tsai; Sell, Timothy C.; Smoliga, James M.; Myers, Joseph B.; Learman, Kenneth E.; Lephart, Scott M. "A Comparison of Physical Characteristics and Swing Mechanics Between Golfers With and Without a History of Low-back Pain." Journal of Orthopaedic & Sports Physical Therapy, Vol 40, Issue 7, 430-438, 2010.

ing a swing, most of you will notice that you have more movement to one side over the other.

Susceptibility to these repeated types of movement can lead the body to create a new motor pattern.[59,60] Over time, you develop a certain threshold; when that is breached for some reason or another, the dysfunction at your pain-free joint starts to breakdown and may cause pain somewhere else.

If you have had an injury or surgery to your right knee, for example, you will shift your weight to your left leg. Very normal. As time passes, your original injury should normalize and heal. However, you may still resort to the same weight shift onto your left leg rather than the right. Because it is a learned habit.

With such sports as tennis and golf, weight shifting to both sides is the big equalizer. You need to be able to do this so you can hit the ball with greater force and speed but at the same time with good control.

You've heard the saying, "Insanity is doing the same thing over and over again and expecting different results." If you continue to resort to the same movement pattern over and over again, and don't take the time to retrain a new strategy, you will get the same results that you've always gotten.

The truth is that the rib cage (thorax), the hip, and the foot are essentially rotational joints. They perform other movements as well, but rotation is what I focus on here. Abnormal foot and ankle mechanics can lead to stress on your hip and back. They can also lead to inefficient hip and pelvic movement patterns. Foot and ankle dysfunction can indeed be the etiology of many pathological conditions. This may lead to postural changes in the body and, as a result of this, ground reaction forces change and can get redirected right up the chain.[61]

---

59   Cohn, Patrick J. The Mental Game of Golf: A Guide to Peak Performance. Taylor Trade Publishing: 2002.

60   Stevens, Joel; Hall, Kellie Green. "Motor Skill Acquisition Strategies for Rehabilitation of Low-back Pain." Journal of Orthopaedic & Sports Physical Therapy, Vol 28, Issue 3, 165-167, 1998.

61   Trachtenberg, George C., "When Lower Extremity Dysfunction Contributes To Back Pain," Podiatry Today, Vol 25, Issue 12, December 2012.

Try serving in tennis while keeping your foot fixed, not allowing it to move at all; you will most certainly feel the strain in your hip and back. In the same way, keeping your right foot fixed, and not allowing it to adapt and rotate in the downswing with golf, will most certainly alter your ability to absorb the ground reaction force. Ultimately, this affects how far you hit the ball.

And who does not want to hit the ball farther?

If you don't allow your back foot to come through when serving in tennis, you will over-flex into your back and shoulder complex. This is not the most desirable scenario.

Story

A very active golfer and tennis player was referred to me by a colleague. At the time of my initial evaluation, he was playing golf more, as it was the summer here in New York City. He had some complaints of right low-back and buttock pain and a secondary complaint of right groin pain.

Sitting, especially in the car, and prolonged standing aggravated his symptoms, as did a long round of golf. His relevant past history consisted of two prior knee surgeries on his right side and a history of a herniated lumbar disc about five years ago. He worked for an international investment bank and was in a seated position for a great deal of his time there. In response to the pain he experienced, his physician had prescribed anti-inflammatories, and he stopped playing golf. Prior to our initial evaluation, he had made little progress.

When he started playing tennis in the fall, he had similar complaints to those he experienced while golfing. These symptoms were aggravated primarily by serving and, more specifically, the follow-through.

In the other golf story (see Chapter 12, "My knee pain is not improving because of tightness in my low-back?") in the book, we talk a lot about the golf swing and how poor mechanics at one joint can trickle up the kinetic chain and cause pain and/or dysfunction somewhere else.

This also happens in tennis. As you can see from the photos at right, there is excessive tension on the back, especially on the follow-through. This is what is supposed to happen. You generate enough force through multiple joints in order to hit the ball well.

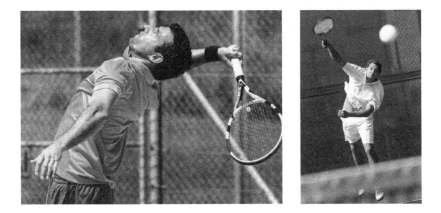

However, when you have excessive mobility in your back, like this patient had, performing this motion over and over again may cause pain and dysfunction unless you have the ability to control it.

He was not tight, so stretching the low-back would not help. Many people think stretching a muscle helps, but if the person is very flexible or if the muscle has been strained over and over again, as was the case here, stretching will make it worse. Think about an acute hamstring strain. The last thing you want to do is stretch.

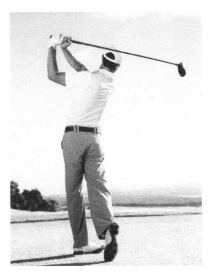

This exaggerated movement also happens in golf on the follow-through while the right hip, torso, and legs are rotating to the left.

What causes that extra flexibility? Is it genetic? Or is it a posture that, when adopted on a continual basis, tends to overstretch certain muscles of the back, which then becomes the norm?

What I Found

Using an integrated total body approach, a few things jumped out at me during the initial evaluation. I like to look at a person's standing posture just to get an idea of where the starting point is, so to speak. This is their baseline. Standing was an issue for him, and it gave me an idea of how he held himself without any load or dynamic movement.

If there are things I find here and I don't find them in other positions, I focus more on the findings in the activities that are relevant for the patient. Since sitting was one of the activities, I looked at his squat to start off. Remember, to get to a sitting position, you have to squat first.

The squat revealed a restriction in his right hip, which prevented him from achieving an optimal hip position when he sat. When he squatted, he seemed to turn his trunk to the left. This also overstressed the right side of his low-back, which reproduced the all-too-familiar pain he felt while sitting.

So where was the source of the pain—the hip, the low-back, or some other part of his body?

I also had him bend his right hip while sitting in order to confirm my belief—that the movement did indeed have an effect on his lower back (see photo below). What he did was to lean or "sit" into the right side of his back, in essence giving into the increased mobility there. This also reproduced his symptoms. This was the strategy his nervous system chose for that particular movement.

As you can see from the photo, when you have limited ability to flex the hip, you will compensate at the low-back. When the hip doesn't move well, the next joint that picks up the slack is generally the low-back.

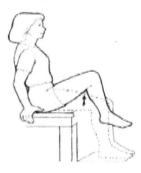

Is this inability from weak abdominals, weak hip flexors, or just a stiff hip? Or could it be from something else far from the hip that was influencing his ability to lift his leg?

Whatever it was, he compensated in the same place. In order to differentiate the source, I played one area off of the other until he was able to squat, sit, and lift his leg without compensation.

I initially determined that his hip was the prime cause for his low-back pain in sitting. I believe that after all the knee surgeries, he had increased tone and overuse in his right quadriceps and adductor muscles, causing altered biomechanics at the hip. After knee surgery, it is quite normal to rehab and strengthen the knee; oftentimes, it is the rehabbed knee that becomes stronger and more dominant. That was the case with this patient.

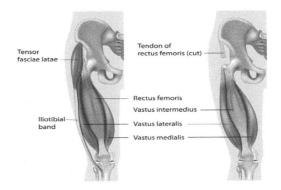

As you can see from the photo above, the anterior muscles of the thigh, such as the rectus femoris (quadricep), tensor fascia latae, and the adductor (not pictured), all attach to the hip and pelvis and will influence the biomechanics and control when they are overworked. This over-recruitment causes increased muscle tone and will influence the hip's ability to move optimally. Once again, your nervous system hard at work!

There is one another component that was affecting the patient's ability to sit and also recover from a long day of golf. As his ability to sit improved, he started to play more golf. The increased left trunk rotation, noted in the squat previously, now became dominant as he played more golf. This caused him problems while he played.

Remember that, for him, this was his path of least resistance. The right side of his low-back was the victim. Since golf is primarily a sport of rotations, one can easily see how this can happen. Once the mechanics at his hip were corrected, this over-rotation became more apparent and dominant.

What Worked

I like to use the term *movement therapy* as well as the word *treatment*. After all, physical therapists are the experts in movement dysfunction.

The patient's hip was treated with a variety of techniques. Some of these included:

- Manual therapy techniques, such as joint mobilization, to decrease the tone in his thigh (clinical experience)

- Soft-tissue release to the muscles in front of his thigh, the rectus femoris as well as the adductor

- Taping to the ribcage to control the rotation while he performed certain exercises.[62]

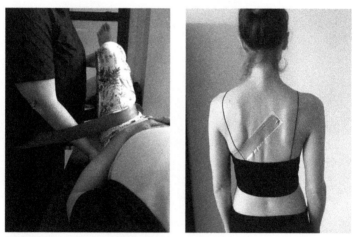

Joint Mobilization for the Hip

- Other techniques included prolonged quad stretching (a twenty-second stretch will not cut it here). In order to effectively decrease the tone in these muscles, it was necessary to stretch for a longer period of time, up to sixty seconds.[63] Please see page 157 for a photo of this stretch.

---

62   Lee, Diane and Lee, Linda Joy (LJ). *Discover Physio Series*, Vancouver, B.C., 2012.

63   Houglum, Peggy. *Therapeutic Exercise for Musculoskeletal Injuries, 4th Edition*. Human Kinetics: 2016.

- Corrective exercise to help him sit properly with an aligned hip. This included all-fours sit-backs (pictured below) with his right hip in external rotation. This was necessary at the beginning so he could seat his hip properly.

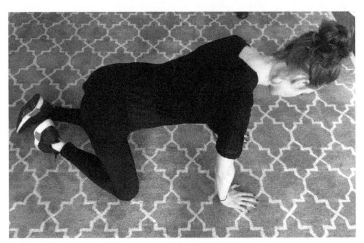

Note the position of the right leg, this puts the right hip in external rotation

- We also did squats with verbal and visual cueing to relax the muscles of the hip. We then progressed to squats with right rotation to reinforce a better movement pattern.

- We also did some lower trunk rotation with upper body rotation to train certain movements that were relevant to golf.

Another great functional move is shown on the next page (ball throws to the right). This really helps control the rotational impairment that he had while working on a stable weight shift.

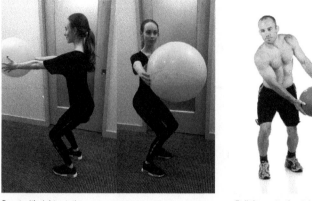

Squat with right rotation   Ball throws to the right

Your treatment options are limitless if you tap into your creativity and make it relevant to the patient.

Positive Results

- Return to golf

- Ability to play better

- Knowledge of what he can do if this happens again

- An empowered patient

- An understanding that if his low-back hurts, it does not mean that the *cause* of the problem is the low-back

- A "think-out-of-the-box" mentality

Tennis

This person started to play tennis again throughout the fall season. He started to experience a similar issue in his low-back when he played, but it was generally the service motion that bothered him. What was really interesting here was that his *right foot* was the source of the problem now, rather than his hip.

You need to develop effective lower body force and energy transfer up the kinetic chain when you serve. When I evaluated his service motion, instead of effectively pushing off with his back right foot, which requires some supination and a bit of a push off, he collapsed his arch and had to get the extra forward motion from his back, which was already strained. Once again, the path of least resistance.

You cannot push off and get the forward motion you need without an effective lever to push from. I ended up releasing some of the muscles in his foot, taping it into a bit more supination. In my lingo, we call it a "navicular lift or sling," to provide some support to the arch.

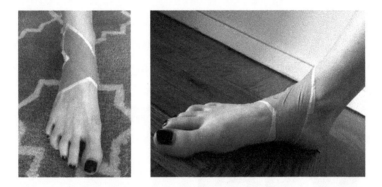

He felt much better with the tape, so he ended up getting some "off-the-shelf" inner soles to wear while he played, and he played well.

I include this in his story, as it really shows the power of a good clinical evaluation. Don't assume that if your low-back hurts that the source for the pain is the same across all activities. A lot of times, it is. But in this case, it wasn't, especially when it comes to sports performance.

Your **nervous system** is **key** to getting rid of your pain

Chapter 5

Really? My **hip pain** comes from an old **abdominal scar**?

Did you know that your hip pain could be caused by scar tissue from an appendectomy?

Did you know that a prior appendectomy could be a factor in your hip pain and your inability to turn, sit, or squat properly?

Truth

Sometimes, old surgical scar tissue can cause new pain and problems. Post-operative intra-abdominal adhesions occur in the majority of people who undergo abdominal surgery. This is an unfortunate truth, and it is often overlooked, especially when it is chronic.

A large percentage of people can develop chronic pain as a result of these adhesions.[64,65] A scar is an area of fibrous tissue that replaces skin after an injury or surgery. Adhesions are bands of this fibrous tissue that form between the organs and these tissues. They form when inflammation occurs on the surface of the abdominal organs or the lining of the abdominal cavity.

---

64   Wong, Yui Y; Smith, Ryan W. Koppenhaver, Shane. "Soft Tissue Mobilization to Resolve Chronic Pain and Dysfunction Associated With Postoperative Abdominal and Pelvic Adhesions: A Case Report." Journal of Orthopaedic & Sports Physical Therapy, Vol 45, Issue 12, 1006-1016, 2015

65   Van RIjckevorsei, Dagmar; de Vries, Marjan; Schreuder, Luuk TW; Wilder-Smith, Oliver HG; van Goor, Harry. Risk factors for chronic postsurgical abdominal and pelvis pain. Pain Management, Vol. 5, Issue 2, 107-116, March 2015.

Scarring is a natural part of the healing process. Without getting into too much detail regarding the composition of scar tissue, suffice it to say that this tissue is composed of collagen, just like the original tissue it replaces. However, it is formed differently. Over time, it can get bound down and restrict movement. This, of course, varies amongst surgical procedures.

Abdominal adhesions, or scar tissue that forms between the abdominal tissue and organs, were an important factor in this patient's presentation. The appendix is on the lower right section of your abdomen; if there is scar tissue from a prior appendix surgery, it could limit your movement.

That is why it is so important to get a patient's full history in the initial evaluation. Patients often say to me, "I had this surgery, but it is not relevant," Trust me; it is *all* relevant. Always allow the medical provider to be the judge of its relevancy.

I'll bet you are thinking, "An appendix scar—are you kidding me?" Actually, no I am not. Different causes, similar symptoms. Remember?

Tightness and restriction in the front of your abdomen, whether from abdominal surgery or a constant breath-holding strategy, can limit your trunk rotation and possibly even your ability to bend backwards. This is particularly relevant for dancers and golfers, as well as tennis players. However, tennis players can compensate a bit more with their feet.

If you get one thing from this book, I want you to get this—everyone is different. That's why the same treatment will not work for everyone.

Cookie-cutter prescriptions are lame and lazy, as are cookie-cutter diagnoses. Think hip pain, back pain, etc. These terms are not diagnostic and do not tell you what and where the source of the pain is.

Furthermore, what if you have no pain? Another reason you would seek a physical therapist's help could be, for example, to treat your endurance (i.e., an inability and weakness to push through your legs while running up a hill). Again, physical therapists should be the frontline defense for any pain and/or movement-related concerns in the body.

Story

A patient of mine wanted to return to dance, but she was unable to dance properly due to lower back and hip pain. Every time she tried to step backwards and turn to the right, her right hip would hurt, especially in dances similar to the rhumba. She also had problems while sitting and turning in the same direction (to the right).

Walking was not as problematic because 1) we don't walk backwards, and 2) although we do rotate when we walk, it was not enough to aggravate her symptoms. In addition, research shows that you alter your walking speed, as well as your movement patterns, and tend to disassociate your pelvis and thorax when you are in pain.[66]

As you can see from the photo below, stepping back and turning are moves integral to dance.

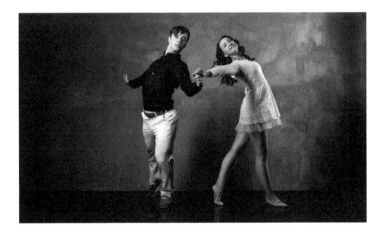

Sitting can be a problem for many people, and the causes are as numerous as the people themselves. We do not function in straight planes; we function in at least three dimensions. Rotation is one of them and takes place in the transverse plane.

---

66   Selles, RW; Wagenaar, RC; Smit TH; Wuisman, PI. "Disorders in trunk rotation during walking in patients with low-back pain: a dynamical systems approach." Clinical Biomechanics, Vol 16, Issue 3, 175-181, Mar 2001.

Sitting may be sedentary, but if you think about it, you do move while seated. We are always reaching to pick up the phone or turning to view our computer screen if it is on one side of the desk. This type of setup creates a bias to either side, for sure. Sitting for hours on end with no break can also cause all sorts of other problems.[67,68]

Being able to move freely while sitting is important. As you can see below, full rotation to the right certainly requires some ease of movement in the front of the trunk.

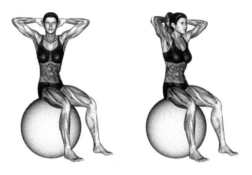

What I Found

My assessment revealed that the source of the problem was in the patient's thorax (the area of the body between the neck and lower back), but it wasn't from joint stiffness. It was from a lack of movement control.

As I have mentioned in other sections of this book, the type of evaluation I perform is based on what type of activity is relevant or meaningful to you. I assess what you can't do or what you want to be able to do and cannot currently.

67   Dunstan, David W.; Howard, Bethany; Healy, Genevieve N.; Owen, Nevile. "Too much sitting – A health hazard." Diabetes Research and Clinical Practice, Vol 97, Issue 3, 368-376. Sept 2012.

68   Evans, Rhian E.; Fawole, Henrietta O.; Sheriff, Stephanie A.; Dall, Philippa M.; Grant, Margaret; Ryan, Cormac G. "Point-of-Choice Prompts to Reduce Sitting Time at Work." American Journal of Preventive Medicine, Vol 43, Issue 3, 293-297, Sept 2012.

In this case, I evaluated both the patient's step back right as well as her squat. Keep in mind that you get to a seated position from a squat.

When she turned to the right and stepped back, the pull of the scar tissue from the appendectomy was causing her to lose balance and use muscles that were inappropriate, which resulted in a lack of movement control as well as hip and back pain. The muscles that I found to be the main culprits in this case were in the front of her abdomen. Clearly, this situation was not ideal. The greatest amount of rotation generally takes place in the mid-back or thorax, not in the lower back.

Her hip certainly was restricted, but it was not from a tight joint or tight hip flexors. This patient was hypermobile, meaning that she had loose ligaments and joints that move in excess of the normal range of motion.

She had physical therapy previously, which focused on strengthening certain muscles of her hip. She did not experience much relief with that type of treatment plan. This revelation did not surprise me, as her hip joint was not the cause of the problem.

Your provider can intervene all day long at the point of your symptomatic area, and if that is not the real source of the problem, then you are wasting your time and money. Her hip was the compensation here. The body takes the path of least resistance, they say, and because she was flexible in her hips, the body took that route.

Our minds and our bodies are very smart; they figure out a strategy to get the job done and move. This workaround develops a motor map in our brains, and when we move a certain way repetitively, such as in dancing or golf, our brain automatically adapts to this type of pattern.[69] Although the squat did not involve rotation like the rhumba, it did reveal a similar impairment. Every time the patient squatted, her trunk shifted to the right.

I was not sure why she did this, but she did. I hypothesized after evaluating her that the pull in the front of the abdomen caused her to shift her center of mass to the right side. Since her surgery was many years ago, this was a learned movement pattern that had to be unlearnt.

---

69   Bilalić, Merim et al. "Editorial: Neural Implementation of Expertise." *Frontiers in Human Neuroscience* 9 (2015): 545. *PMC*. Web. 18 May 2017.

What Worked

For the patient's primary intervention, I addressed the issues that surfaced during the initial assessment and devised a strategy to target each area of concern.

What I did

- Release and mobilization of scar tissue

- Specific movement control exercises

- Abdominal release techniques

- Taping of the right middle ribs to provide control for new movement pattern[70]

- Movement program that encouraged more lateral (side-to-side) control along with improved step back and rotation

At the outset, I focused on the necessary release and mobilization of the scar tissue and specific movement control exercises. Some of the abdominal release techniques I used were derived from French osteopath, Jean-Pierre Barral.[71] Once this was done, I taped the patient's right ribs so as to provide her with some control while her new movement pattern was being retrained. This is important, as oftentimes we feel relief after a treatment intervention, but then the carryover

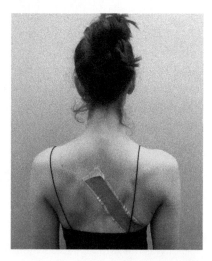

is poor, because we resort to an old movement pattern. With taping, this enables proper movement retraining without the old pattern dominating.

---

70   Lee, Diane and Lee, Linda Joy (LJ), *Discover Physio Series*, Vancouver, B.C., 2012.

71   Barral, Jean Pierre. Mercier, Pierre. Visceral Manipulation. Eastland Press, Revised Edition: 2006.

Since this was such a chronic problem, the release and taping were done every treatment session initially. We also did some techniques to increase the movement at the hip joints because of the chronicity of her problem, but this constituted about 30 percent of the treatment plan, as this was not the cause of her problem.

I performed other manual treatment techniques as well, but the explanation of these is beyond the scope of this book. Suffice it say, these were hands-on specific techniques local to the cause of the problem.

Movement Program

- Side-stepping exercises to give more lateral (side-to-side) control

- Step-back lunges with rotation

- Specific yoga postures to open up the abdomen

- Strength training specific to the patient's issues

Her original exercise plan (or "movement program," as I like to call it) included side-stepping exercises to give her more lateral control. This is of course a necessary component to dance. We later progressed to step backs, step-back lunges and then step-back lunges with rotation, which were similar to her dance moves.

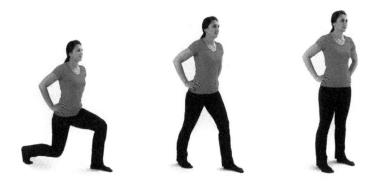

If we wanted to incorporate and progress to a more "gym-like" routine, she could have done step-back lunges in a star-like pattern (stepping out at 45, 60, 75, and 90 degree angles, etc.) which would simulate the step back and rotation technique seen in dancing. These exercises were specific to her problem and reinforced control in the movements she needed to strengthen. Giving her front lunges would not have worked in this case, as they would not have challenged her control and were irrelevant to her.

If you wanted another exercise to progress this type of controlled movement, you could try the same movement on the Pilates Reformer, incorporating the strength, balance, and agility required in the practice of Pilates.

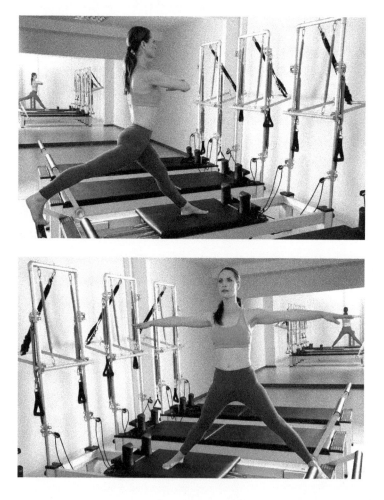

This movement could also be done sideways on the Reformer. It is all about training control here.

Additional Treatment

I prescribed specific yoga postures, such as the triangle pose, to open up and stretch the right side of the patient's abdomen. These were done to retrain a new motor pattern in her brain. I initially had her keep the tape on for all exercises, and then I weaned her off the taping once her control was better established.

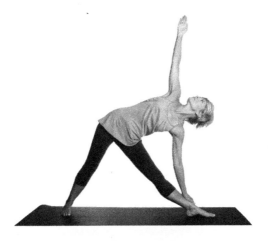

What is important to note is that these movements were *specific* to her problem. There has been a lot of research done regarding motor control training and its importance in a rehab program.[72,73]

Strength training is also important and has a place in rehab. However, with chronic issues that have not gotten better, such as in the case of this patient, an in-depth assessment regarding muscle imbalances is always warranted. What you often will find is that certain muscle groups are *inhibited*, not weak.

72   Nijs, Jo; Cagnie, Barbara; Rouseel, Nathalie A.; Dolphens, Mieke; Van Oosterwijck, Jessica; Danneels, Lieven. "A Modern Neuroscience Approach to Chronic Spinal Pain: Combining Pain Neuroscience Education With Cognition-Targeted Motor Control Training." Physical Therapy Journal of the APTA, Vol 94, Issue 5, 730-738. May 2014.

73   Winter, David A. Biomechanics and Motor Control of Human Movement, 4th Edition. Wiley: 2009.

The purpose of specific controlled movements in physiotherapy is to wake up those muscle groups. Using your brain to control the movement will in part do this.

These are just a few of the movements that I included in her program. As long as you are creative, the potential for a varied and fun rehab program is endless!

Positive Results

- A return to dancing
- Much improved control of movement in her thorax
- Increased right leg stability
- Empowerment and understanding of how to prevent and manage her condition

Imagining
movement
is almost
as good as
doing it

Really? My **hip** continues to bother me because of an issue with my **pelvis** and **foot**?

Did you know that if the labrum is not the source of your groin pain, the surgery to repair a torn labrum in your hip will often not be completely successful?

Truth

Just because you are looking down the barrel of an MRI that states unequivocally that you have a torn labrum in your hip, this does not mean that you need a surgical procedure to repair it.

Does this surprise you?

This is the ultimate in frustration. However, it is important to know that a lot of people have torn labrums and function just fine. On the contrary, there are others such as baseball player Alex Rodriguez, Olympic Sprinter Tyson Gay, or singer Lady Gaga, who, because of the nature of their professions, decided to have surgery because it was affecting their performance.

The hip is a rotary joint and functions in more than one plane. The labrum is a ring of cartilage that lines the hip joint. It provides stability to the joint.

Athletes who participate in sports such as soccer, ice hockey, golf, and baseball are prone to these issues. Structural abnormalities in the hip have a high correlation with labral tears.[74,75] This may have been the case with the patient in this story.

There are many sources of hip pain. At times, the labrum is the poor victim. For example, if you injure your right foot, the normal response is to offload that leg and increase the weight on your left leg. This may create a shift in your body. It becomes almost a fixed response. This can affect how you recruit certain muscles, especially on the side where you are putting more weight. In addition, these compensations may lead to abnormal muscle and joint mechanics down the road.

To follow this injury to many years later, an old right ankle sprain suddenly produces a left hip issue because of all the years of abnormal compensation. The body adapts well until it has reached its tolerance or buckle point. That is when you begin to notice aches and stiffness in your hip because it has reached its limit of adaptability.

The point here is that you may have a torn labrum in your hip from an old unrelated injury. Though an MRI may show a torn labrum, the real cause of the problem may be far from your hip. Many practitioners stop at the hip when, in fact, it may not be the real source of the problem.

If your pain is chronic, you may end up having surgery in the end and may even feel better. However, you could still have some groin pain while

The Hip Joint

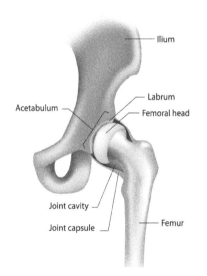

Ilium
Labrum
Femoral head
Acetabulum
Joint cavity
Joint capsule
Femur

74   McCormick, Frank; Nwachukwu, Benedict U.; Alpaugh, Kyle; Martin, Scott D. "Predictors of Hip Arthroscopy Outcomes for Labral Tears at Minimum 2-Year Follow-up: The Influence of Age and Arthritis." Arthroscopy: The Journal of Arthroscopic and Related Surgery, Vol 28, Issue 10, 1359-1364. Oct 2012.

75   Hosnijeh, F. Saberi; Versteeg, M.; Smelle, J.; Hoffman, A.; Uitterlinden, A.G.; Agricola, R.; Oei, E.H.; Waarsing, J.H.; Bierrna-Zeinstra, S.M.; van Meurs, J.B. "The Shape of the Hip Joint as a risk factor for osteoarthritis." Osteoarthritis and Cartilage Journal, Vol 24, Supp 1, S21-S22, April 2016.

walking. Why? Because ultimately the hip was not the original source of the problem or is not the source of the problem now. You won't get 100 percent relief until the major cause of the pain is corrected.

Story

One of my patients had surgery to repair a torn labrum in her left hip. She had tried rehab pre-operatively in another state to see if she could avoid the procedure, but ultimately she had the surgery done. I saw her for the first time several months after the surgery was completed. She had begun rehab in her home state after the surgery. Since she did not live in New York City, the visits needed to coincide with her trips to New York. Prior to her surgery, she had also received two cortisone injections in her hip, which actually worsened her problem.

When I spoke with her over the phone before her initial evaluation, she was still on crutches nearly four months after surgery. She was obviously anxious to get off the crutches. Her main complaints were groin pain and a "tightness" in the front part of her left thigh, both of which were aggravated by walking. She had an additional complaint of lateral hip pain and had difficulty lifting her left leg as in the photo below.

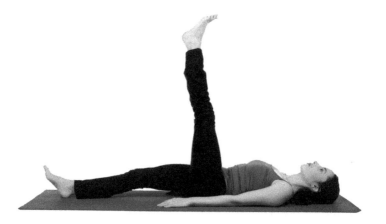

This is called an active straight leg raise and is a fairly common exercise prescribed to patients with knee or hip pain. As you can see from the image below of some gait patterns, there are many joints, from our feet to our arms and torso, that need to move in order for us to walk with some semblance of ease—ease is relative, of course. There are some people who just want to walk ten blocks, while there are others who want to walk three miles. Whether it is ten blocks or three miles, the mechanics are the same. Simply speaking, the hip moves forward when we swing our leg through, and it extends backward when it is behind us.

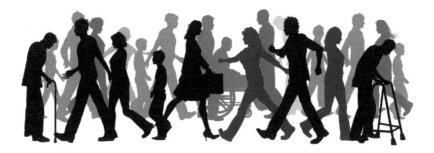

Imagine that you have surgery to correct a labral tear or that you have pain in the front of the hip or in the groin. Your chief complaint is that you are unable to walk without hip pain or a tightness in your thigh. Some common compensations for this include swinging the leg forward and inward, almost as if you are turning your hip and leg in. Other compensations include shortening your step length because of tight hip flexors.[76]

Many of these compensations are subconscious in the sense that we do not realize we are doing them; however, the body is smart and it operates in an effort to avoid pain when it can. Over time, this type of gait pattern becomes our norm, our compensation, our crutch. In my clinical experience, these compensations are what need to be addressed first for chronic problems, if in fact they are the cause of the problem.

What I Found

Since walking was the main problem—specifically, putting the left leg forward—that is what I assessed. I also looked at her straight leg raise to see how she could load her leg in an unweighted position. Since she had

---

76 Clinical Experience

a problem with this, it was important to her that it be incorporated into the evaluation.

I evaluated her stepping forward as this, of course, is an integral part of walking. When she stepped forward with her left foot, her hip and pelvis turned excessively to the right, as if she were leading with her left shoulder.

When you take a step forward with your left foot, your pelvis is supposed to turn to the right, but hers went WAY right. It was almost as if she was turning her whole body to the right, overactivating the muscles of her inner left thigh and practically shifting all the weight onto her right leg, which was behind her. Why did she do this?

There are many reasons why the body does what it does. That is your nervous system at its best. But with her, I believe it was a strategy of convenience, as the body takes the path of least resistance. You keep doing the same thing over and over, and the body thinks it is normal and does very little to change it until a buckle point is reached. Or in her case, a labral tear and a subsequent surgical procedure to repair it.

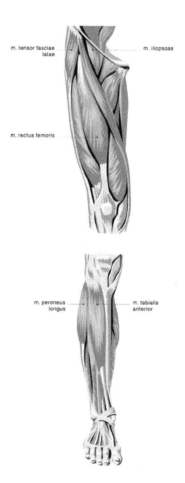

Her left hip and pelvis (which was the hip operated on), was turning in, or *internally rotating* in my lingo, an excessive amount. Because of this strategy, she was over-activating the anterior muscles of her hip, namely the tensor fasciae latae, psoas, and the rectus femoris. Additionally, she was putting an excessive amount of weight onto her left foot, not only over-activating the front of her thigh but also the muscles in and around her lower leg and foot.

I believe that over time this over-activation was one of the causes of the tight feeling she was having in the front of her thigh. But what was causing the groin pain and this tightness to persist?

I played one area off of the other, trying to facilitate a better movement pattern for her when she stepped forward with her left leg. I did this manually, making modifications to her pelvis and hip for starters. Sometimes this is hard to do, but you do the best you can. The best result was when I supported her pelvis. This means that she had the least amount of tightness and pain. Note that this is not the hip joint.

ANATOMY OF THE PELVIS

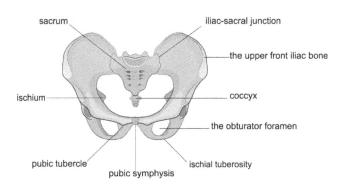

She had similar complaints when she performed the straight leg raise. My evaluation revealed similarly that when I gave her support to the back of her pelvis, she was able to lift her leg much easier and without complaints of tightness or pain.[77, 78, 79]

77   Stuge, Britt. "The automatic pelvic floor muscle response to the active straight leg raise in pelvic girdle pain and matched controls." Manual Therapy, Vol 18, Issue 4, 327-332, Aug 2013.

78   Lee, Diane G. The Pelvic Girdle: An Integration of Clinical Expertise and Research, 4th edition. Churchill Livingstone: 2010.

79   Vleeming, Andry. Movement, Stability & Lumbopelvic Pain: Integration of Research and Therapy, 2nd Edition. Churchill Livingstone: 2007.

The relief she experienced with pelvic support meant that she may have been over-activating certain muscles at the front of her pelvis and perhaps underusing the muscles of the back of her pelvis.[80]

The *main takeaway* here is that the actual hip joint was not the cause of her problem (much to her relief!). Imagine having hip surgery and then being told that the hip is still the problem.

I only had a couple of treatment sessions with her before she went back to her home state.

---

80   Bruno, Paul A.; Goertzen, Dale A.; Millar, David P. "Patient-reported perception of difficulty as a clinical indicator of dysfunctional neuromuscular control during the prone hip extension test and active straight leg raise test." Manual Therapy, Vol 19, Issue 6, 602-607, Dec 2014.

What Worked

As I discussed previously, I found that she was over-activating the anterior muscles of her hip and thigh and reproducing her symptoms. In addition, upon further assessment she was shifting her trunk to the left and turning her foot in a way that was not optimal (more on that later).

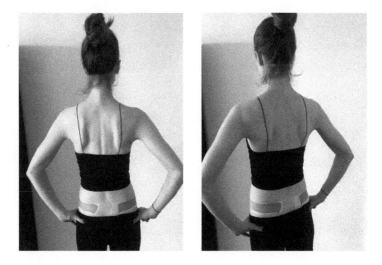

What I did

- Released some of the muscles pulling on the pelvis

- Taping of pelvis posteriorly[81]

- Walking backwards to engage muscles in the back of her pelvis and legs, mimicking the taped pelvic support

- Had the patient begin using a pelvic belt[82] to replace the taping

- Introduced a bent leg raise while taped to retrain her brain in that movement pattern. As the active straight leg raise was difficult, I had her perform it with a bent leg to start.

---

81   Lee, Diane and Lee, Linda Joy (LJ). *Discover Physio Series*, Vancouver, B.C., 2012.

82   https://www.dianelee.ca/article-si-belt-compressor.php

As stated above, I released some of the muscles that were pulling on the pelvis and taped her pelvis posteriorly (see photo). I then had the patient do some walking backwards, which was fairly easy for her with no pain or tightness. Walking backwards also engaged muscles in the back of her pelvis and legs, which exactly mimicked the type of pelvic support she received while her pelvis was taped. I eventually ended up getting her a pelvic belt that replaced the tape.

To complete her treatment, I had her do a bent leg raise while she was taped in order to retrain her brain and get her leg used to lifting with different mechanics (since it was taped). Performing the leg lift with the leg bent initially lessened the force on the hip.

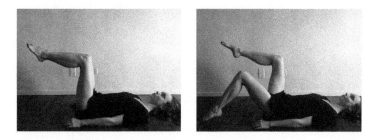

If yoga is your thing, you can try some of these poses to open up the front and sides of the pelvis. Ultimately, we want to train a new movement pattern.

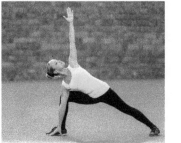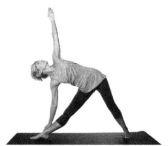

Since the patient was only in New York City for two days, I saw her immediately the next day. She reported that her walking was better with the pelvic belt on. I did a short reassessment of her stepping forward and noticed something with her foot, which I had seen prior but did not focus on because it was not the prime source of her problem.

My concern was that her foot was losing control as she stepped forward on her left foot (increasing the pronation). I performed a similar evaluation, albeit a shorter one, with the focus on the foot. Pronation is a normal component of the gait cycle, but in her case it was occurring excessively and early. In and out itself, not a problem for most people.

But when someone has a long history like this, it is often very common to find other secondary issues that are contributing to the problem. This was the case with her foot. Without getting into too much detail here in this story, she had muscle imbalances and joint restrictions in her foot that were additionally contributing to her hip problem. When these were treated, her stepping forward was even better.

If she lived in New York City and could come in for regular treatment, I may not have looked at the foot so quickly in the initial sessions. But I wanted her to go home with a comprehensive treatment plan so that she could incorporate my suggestions before she came in again, which was weeks to months later.

The second takeaway here is that your therapist should always be reassessing you and remain on the lookout for other sources of your problems as your rehab progresses or if you plateau.

I'm happy to share that this patient is now managing on her own, using her new strategies. She occasionally checks in with me virtually. However, she is off her crutches, her standing and walking are a lot better, and she can now lift her leg up easily.

The reason I selected this particular story is this: If you continue to have persistent symptoms, even after surgery, it's not that the surgical procedure went wrong. It is possible that there is another source to your problem. I strongly advise you to seek out the advice of a licensed professional to address your symptoms and concerns. Don't give up!

X-rays and scans **do not show pain**

Chapter 7

Really? My sacro-iliac joint hurts because of poor foot control?

Did you know that sacro-iliac (SI) joint and posterior pelvic pain can be primarily caused by a dysfunction in your foot?

Truth

As you will see in both pelvic/SI joint stories, pelvic pain can be caused by a structure in your body far away from your pelvis. And in this patient's story, the primary source is the foot.

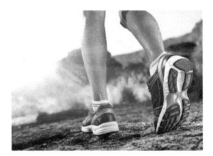

The foot is the main lever for push off during gait. It assists in weight transfer as we move forward and is a key component for balance. If there is a dysfunction in the foot, but it is pain-free, we often ignore it, as we do not know anything is "wrong."

Until we try to run or walk uphill, for example. Then something else hurts. You know the old saying that when the foot hits the ground, everything changes—literally. The power of the kinetic chain is no more powerful than it is here.

Dysfunction in one body part can set up a chain reaction in your body and usually we can compensate for it, depending on age, flexibility, and fitness level. The older we get, the harder it is for us to compensate. The more flexible we are, the easier it is to compensate and athletes are the best compensators of all. Your nervous system adjusts to your changing movement patterns.

The foot is the foundation of our body and our connection to the earth, and a chronic problem there may induce stresses on other muscles and joints up the leg into the pelvis, low-back, and even higher.

As a matter of fact, an article written in *Arthritis Care and Research* on the influence of foot position on the spine and pelvis showed that changes in foot position also led to significant changes in pelvic position. You may say, "Cause or effect?" Either way, they have some relationship.[83]

Having a global approach like this is a critical aspect to successful rehab. Without this, you run the risk of not discovering the true source of your problem or, at the very least, not finding a long-term solution to your pain.

When you have activities that require endurance and/or increased loading forces, the kinetic chain (including the brain!) and its relevant biomechanics become more important. For example, when someone jumps repeatedly—like a dancer or a volleyball player—a dysfunctional foot plays a much more significant role. However, it is not just biomechanics; it is the integration of your nervous system with the dynamic strategies that you use for movement (or that we each use to move).

Everybody is different as to how one body part affects another part. This is the compensation that I spoke about earlier. When you are performing a high-level activity, and that differs for everyone, compensation becomes increasingly harder.

Another study looked at the effects of calcaneal eversion (think of pronation at the heel) on three-dimensional kinematics of the hip, pelvis, and thorax while standing on one leg. This study looked at different arch heights as well as different positions of the rear foot. They concluded that changing heel position does affect the kinematics of the thorax, hip, and pelvis.[84] Simply put, if you change your foot position it will have an effect on the joints above. And that certainly was the case with the patient in this story.

---

83   Betsch, M; Schneppendahl, J; Dor, L; Jungbluth, P; Windolf, J; Thelen, S; Hakimi, M; Rapp, W; Wild, M. "Influence of foot positions on the spine and pelvis." Arthritis Care Research, Vol 63, Issue 12, Dec 2011.

84   Yi, Jaehoon. "The effects of increased unilateral and bilateral calcaneal eversion on pelvic and trunk alignment in standing position," Physical Therapy Rehabilitation Science, Vol 5, Issue 84: 8, June 2016.

> " It is not just biomechanics; it is the integration of your nervous system with the dynamic strategies that you use for movement. "

Story

Several months ago, a physiotherapist came to see me from out of town. She had been experiencing longstanding left posterior pelvic pain as well as a "tight" feeling and a "lack of power" in her left hamstring. She had been on a few physiotherapy courses where they attempted to find the source of her problem.

She had a hard time walking long distances, running, and running up hills. Also, when she did a forward bend as in a yoga posture, she "felt it" in her hamstring. Going up stairs, she felt like she lacked power in her leg. Was it a lack of strength or just an inhibited muscle? Sometimes when we feel "weak," or lack power with certain movements, it could be that the muscle tendon unit is in an inefficient position to provide stability during certain activities, rather than a muscle that lacks strength.

The patient had sprained her left ankle in 2009 while she was running, ran a half marathon in November of the same year, played soccer which aggravated her hamstring, and started a yoga teacher training course at that time as well. As is the case with some of the more chronic and complicated patients, she had been to many practitioners, other physical therapists, chiropractors, and osteopaths with minimal to no relief.

She was getting frustrated with her lack of progress. It is important to address this frustration at the onset. What a therapist does or does not address can alter how a patient feels. This can't be more true than in patients who have unsolved pain. A recent article in *The Manual Therapy Journal* discussed how physical therapists may need to spend more time educating their patients on the cognitive and emotional issues that factor into prolonged pain and reassure them that it is common and in no way delegitimizes their pain.[85]

---

85   Van Wilgen, P; Roussel, N; Leysen, M; Beetsma, A; Kuppens, K; Nijs, J. "Do Therapists Understand the Perceptions and Health Behavior of Patients with Chronic Musculoskeletal Pain." Manual Therapy Journal, Vol 25, E65, Sept 2016.

Asking a person how they cope with their pain is vital in the first visit because it gives a glimpse into how they manage their symptoms, if at all. Some people have a healthy relationship with pain and some do not. You're thinking, "Healthy relationship with pain? What's that?" A healthy relationship with pain is when you realize that your pain is there for a reason to protect you in acute situations. Think acute ankle sprain or falling down and hitting your knee cap. Ouch! And as you get older, some aches and pains that come and go are natural.

It is the *persistent pain* that tests us. It challenges us to open our minds and hearts to what role pain does play in our life. There is a saying that goes, "When you have pain, and constantly think about it, you have more pain." That is how your brain works. What you focus on you get. Period.

This patient had a healthy relationship with pain, and although she was frustrated, she was hopeful. And that's what you want.

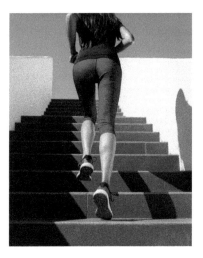

You can see from the picture at left that the foot is the lever for the push up the hill. The foot is not the only piece that works in this situation, however. The hip and knee certainly do their share of the work. And this work translates all the way up the chain, even to the arms and shoulders.

The patient had her pelvis (symptomatic area) treated in the past with not much long-term relief. Why? Because the pelvis was the victim in this case. As I have emphasized throughout this book, the symptomatic area is most likely not the PRIMARY cause of the problem, especially when pain is persistent. Though it may be playing a small role, it certainly does not mean it's the lead cause. This dynamic of cause and effect is common in longstanding and persistent pain problems.

What I Found

Since walking and running are different yet similar activities, you have to look at actions that share commonalities with each movement. So naturally, standing on one leg, (aka, one-legged balance) was the first thing I looked at in the initial evaluation. Walking and running both have what is called a single-leg stance phase, where proper balance is crucial to correct, effective movement.

When you stand on one leg, the ground reaction force pulls on your center of mass, such that you have to stabilize the standing leg via muscular action at the hip and elsewhere. If you have problems standing on one leg, whether it is a true balance problem or some muscular pull from above or below that is causing a balance issue, this can usually be ascertained by comparing the normal mechanics for this activity versus what is actually happening with the patient.

If you can't balance well on one leg, then how do you expect to walk and run efficiently? There are many people who have lousy balance and obviously do walk and run fine. But they are compensating somewhere else, and it's only a matter of time until their buckle point or threshold will be reached. They will eventually run out of options. For some people, that may manifest as muscle fatigue or increased energy expenditure during the task or pain.

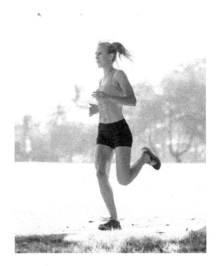

You can see from the photo above that running is a single leg activity and if there were an alteration in the movement of the standing leg, or even the amount of trunk rotation, it would affect the balance. When my patient stood on her left leg, she displayed some shifts in her trunk (thorax), and her left foot was poorly controlled. In layman's terms, she had a harder time stabilizing on that side and used her ankles and upper trunk to help stand upright. Though her thorax and left foot revealed some compensations, her pelvis was fine.

I then played one area off the other to see what made for the best experience for her, where she was better able to stand on one leg. I determined that if I manually corrected her foot (see photo below), she was able to balance a lot better, her pain was decreased, and the compensations displayed in the other areas were diminished.

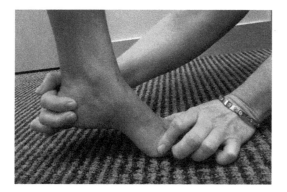

I then further assessed her while she took a step forward with her right foot, such that the left leg was behind. That was her power leg, and the activity where she complained of a lack of power in her left hamstring.

Stepping forward is integral to walking, running, and many other sports and is an excellent way to breakdown the strategies used during the gait cycle.

As you can see on the next page, when we take a step forward, we have to rotate our trunk and pelvis so that we maintain a straight path, so to speak. There should be a counter rotation in your thorax and pelvis—when you step forward with the right foot, your pelvis rotates to the left and your thorax to the right and vice versa.

When she stepped forward with her right foot, she displayed a restriction in her back left foot that was not optimal and her trunk (thorax) rotated to the left, which is the opposite of what should occur. Once again, when we aligned the foot properly, the movement was much improved.

Exercise: You can just try standing and rotating your torso and see how it affects other parts of your body, including the foot.

After the patient's step forward was analyzed thoroughly, I determined that her foot was, again, the prime source of her pelvic pain with walking.

I then wanted to validate her feelings about her hamstring power—or lack thereof. This may seem a lot to do in the evaluation, but bear in mind that she was traveling to New York City from out of town, and I did not have the luxury of waiting for the next treatment session to evaluate it.

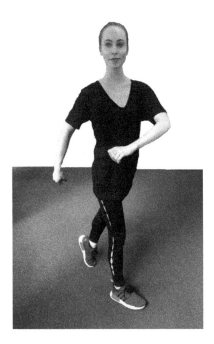

I tested her ability to lift her leg off the table while she was lying on her tummy.[86] This is called prone hip extension and is a great test to use with persistent hamstring strains to determine if the pelvis needs to be addressed.[87,88] As I suspected, her left leg was much harder to lift than the right. I then assessed the impact of the pelvis on her strength, and it was still hard to lift. It has been shown that pelvic compression via the application of a pelvic belt has a facilitative effect on hamstring strength.[89]

86   Lee, Diane G. The Pelvic Girdle: An Integration of Clinical Expertise and Research, 4th edition. Churchill Livingstone: 2010.

87   Ji-Won Kim; Min-Hyeok, Kang; Jae-Seop Oh. "Patients with Low-back Pain Demonstrate Increased Activity of the Posterior Oblique Sling Muscle During Prone Hip Extension." Physical Medicine & Rehab, Vol 6, Issue 5, 400-405, May 2014.

88   Emami, Mahnaz; Arab, Amir Massoud; Ghamkar, Leila. "The activity pattern of the lumbo-pelvis muscles during prone hip extension in athletes with and without hamstring strain injury." International Journal of Sports Physical Therapy, Vol 9, Iss 3, 312-319, May 2014.

89   Arumugan, Ashokan; Milosavijevic, Stephan; Woodley, Stephanie; Sole, Gisela. "Effects of external pelvic compression on isokinetic strength of the thigh muscles in sportsmen with and without hamstring injuries." Journal of Medicine in Science and Sport, Vol 18, Iss 3, 283-288. May 2015

But that was not the case here.

She still displayed the issues in her trunk (thorax), such that when she lifted the leg off the table, in order for her to get more power she 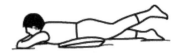 ended up shifting her rib cage to the right to gain more control in the leg. This is common. She also displayed the same twist in her foot while lying prone that she exhibited while performing the step forward.

Once again, when I neutralized her foot, she was able to lift her leg up much more easily. This was also true for the standing forward bend position that she did in yoga. When her foot was modified, she was able to bend forward without feeling her hamstring.

The one consistency that I found throughout all activities was that her foot was the primary source of her problem. In the addendum to this story, we will find that another secondary source needed some attention once the primary cause was treated and she was feeling better.

What Worked

Since the foot was the main issue initially, I started treatment there.

What I did

- Standard soft tissue muscle releases to the foot muscles, including the *anterior tibialis* and *peroneals*

- Manual therapy to her foot

- Taping of rear foot into neutral[90]

- Taught patient to self-mobilize and self-tape

- Exercises, including standing calf stretch with the knee straight and bent on a half foam roll, standing weight shift with a reminder to neutralize her heel, and a stride stance position to work on the power in her left leg

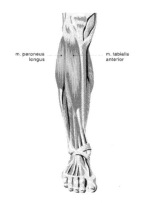

m. peroneus longus   m. tabialis anterior

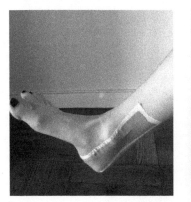

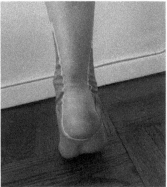

Rear foot taping

90 Lee, Diane and Lee, Linda Joy (LJ). *Discover Physio Series*, Vancouver, B.C., 2012.

I performed standard soft tissue releases to the muscles that were holding the foot in its non-optimal position. These muscles included the *anterior tibialis* and the *peroneals.*

I also taped her rear foot into neutral to help offload the forces going up the leg. In order to give her adequate resources since she was not local, I taught her how to self-mobilize as well as to self-tape.

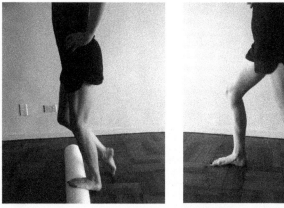

Calf stretch   Stride stance

Other things she had to do included the following: standing calf stretch with the knee straight and bent on a half foam roll (could also do this on a book or towels) and a standing weight shift with a cue to neutralize her heel.

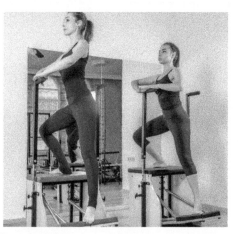

Wunda Box Pushdowns

Once that was mastered, she progressed herself to a stride stance (see photo on previous page) which mimicked the running and walking postures. While performing these exercises, she is made aware of her foot and given cues to help keep it in its optimal position.

Since she was not local, I gave this to her initially and then we kept in touch via email and progressed accordingly. We could have also added the following Pilates and yoga exercises.

One Pilates exercise uses push-downs on the Wunda Box. This simulates the push off of the back left leg while running.

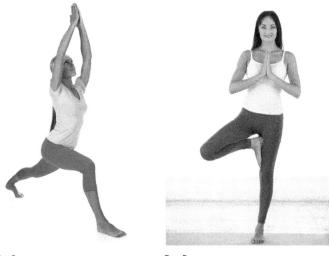

Warrior One   Tree Pose

In this case, we could have used it to increase her hamstring strength to mimic the push through or the propulsion up hills.

We could have done the following yoga postures:

- Warrior One or Warrior Two pose to train the weight shift and push off of the back left foot

- Seated calf raises for foot control

- Tree Pose with cues for the foot to help with balance

- Finally, walking backwards is a great way to train foot control as well.

These are just some examples of what you can do to train the foot in functional postures. There are countless ways to reinforce optimal position and movement of the foot.

Results/Addendum:

She did this fairly religiously for two months and came back to New York City for a follow-up visit. She told me she was feeling much better, walking with the dog was easier, and she was able to power up hills now. Additionally, she shared that her balance was much better. She had also been conscientious with the self-taping and felt that it really helped her.

I performed a reevaluation and found that indeed her foot control was much better. I reassessed the same four movements that we evaluated initially:

- Standing Forward Bend
- One-legged Balance
- Step Forward Right
- Prone Hip Extension (PHE)

I also added a one-legged squat as well as a seated trunk rotation (see page 189). I did this because she wanted to start running again and had not run in a long time. You need trunk rotation to run efficiently, and we do not run with straight legs, so a single-leg mini squat was used to assess her control.

Her one-legged balance and step forward were all fine now. However, when I checked her forward bend, she was feeling a "pull" in the calf instead of the hamstring, and when I checked her ability to lift her left leg up (PHE), it was still harder than the right, but it was easier than the last time.

In both of these movements, she still used her upper trunk to stabilize herself. So when she bent forward or did the prone leg lift, she shifted her trunk to the right. This had happened previously, but when we neutralized the foot, the trunk shift was better, though not totally gone.

In short, when her foot position was modified, all the activities were easier for her, but now we had to address the compensation in her trunk. In the end, when her foot and her thorax (trunk) position were modified together, her left leg was stronger and she was able to bend forward much better.

What I think sometimes gets lost is the ability of your body to adapt to treatment interventions and, most importantly, the ability and willingness of your physical therapist to adapt with you. That is the beauty of the nervous system. It is constantly changing! We often hear things like, "We worked on my foot (knee, back, etc.) and I got much better, but I still can't run (play tennis, etc.)." This is where looking up and down the kinetic chain is so very important.

More often than not, the more load you place on the body, the greater the likelihood that there is a secondary source to your problem. That secondary problem will need to be addressed in order for you to do the activity you long to do. That is why it is vital that you are reassessed if you have hit a plateau; there could be something else lurking that, once addressed, will get you where you want to be.

" Changing someone's movement strategy is the ultimate game changer. "

When I checked her trunk rotation in sitting, she had a limitation to the right. When I checked the one-legged squat on the left, the foot was also not ideal. Remember we don't run with a rigid trunk or straight legs.

Exercise: Try standing on one leg with a little bit of a knee bend and shift your trunk to one side; you will see how that throws your balance off. It is how your nervous system reacts to that loss of balance which is crucial. Do we fall, or does our brain say, "I'll compensate somewhere else, so I don't fall"?

In the end, I progressed her foot program and then added some corrective exercises for her thorax. One of these can be found below. These two components constituted my secondary treatment for her and were ultimately successful in eliminating pain in her SI joint and building up strength in her previously weaker hamstring.

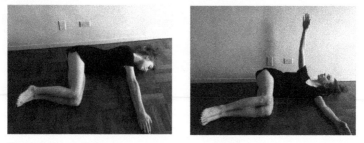

Thoracic Book covers/Openers

I think the ultimate lesson here is that when you have had long-term persistent pain, you need to look at the body from a holistic standpoint. That is, treatment of the whole person, from head to toe, taking into account cognitive and social factors, rather than just the physical symptoms of a disease. In addition, be open to your practitioner working through the different layers to discover what will be the key to a good result for you. Again, everyone is different and a good result for you will be achieved in a uniquely effective way.

Our brain produces opioids **50x more powerful** than an injection

Really? My **sacro-iliac joint** is not getting better because my **abdominal muscles** are overactive?

Did you know that pelvic and SI joint pain can be caused by overactive abdominal muscles?

Truth

Pelvic pain, whether internal or external, can be caused by a structure in your body that is relatively far away from your pelvis.

The pelvis is composed of several joints, viscera, muscles, and ligaments. Additionally, you see below and on the following page that the abdominal muscles are connected to the pelvis and rib cage by nature of their location and attachments.

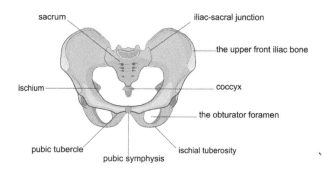

In these images, you can see there are two sides to the pelvis, two innominate bones (top of the "hip bones"), with the sacrum in the middle and the pubic rami in the front. (Not to belabor the anatomy—you can always refer to an anatomy book if you are interested in further study.)

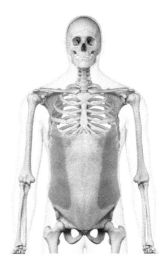

Typically, when referring to their pelvis, patients will point to the sacrum or to the top of the pelvis (or just put their hand on their butt) and say, "I hurt here." Some patients may have pain in their legs as well.

Pelvic pain can be very debilitating, and you owe it to yourself to find someone who can assess and treat it from a holistic mindset and not just manipulate the SI joint because they think it's "gone out." One cannot look at the pelvis without looking at the lumbar spine (low-back) and the hips. These regions make up a functional complex in our bodies and are essential in helping transfer loads from one area to another.

There are many causes to pelvic pain—one can be the low-back, which is the obvious one, but it could also come from inside the pelvic cavity (which would necessitate a referral to a physical therapist who specializes in women's health) or originate from somewhere else. In this case, the pelvic pain came from somewhere else.

The pelvis helps maintain our posture and stability as well as allowing for mobility of other body parts during challenging environments. This is especially true of a dancer, which this particular patient happened to be. In order for a dancer to perform at such a high level doing complex movements repeatedly, there are many control strategies from which to choose. There are also many buckle points, as we call them. They say, "The body takes the path of least resistance," and this is particularly true with a dancer.

Story

A year ago, another health care practitioner referred a patient to me because they had been working with her for some time and the treatment had plateaued. She was referred to me "for another set of eyes," or a second opinion. She was a modern dancer but frequently performed moves that originate in classical ballet.

Her chief complaint was left pelvic/SI joint pain, particularly when she performed an arabesque. When she kicked her left leg back and turned it out while standing "en pointe" on her right leg, she experienced pain on the left side of her pelvis, or SI joint. "It feels jammed," she said.

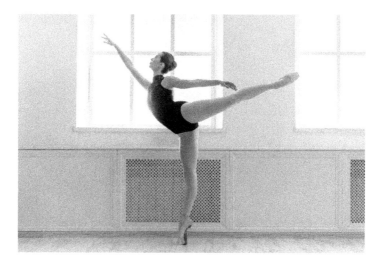

Additionally, she was performing in an opera which required her to maintain certain positions for over an hour (yes, over an hour!). This included sitting with her knees bent (off the ground) and her torso rotated to one side.

Imagine doing this for one hour continuously! As you can imagine, this caused her to develop obvious restrictions in her abdominal muscles, which were ultimately compensated for by her pelvis and other muscles and joints. Because these muscles were so overworked, they limited her trunk rotation. (See page 179 for a photo of these muscles.) When she had to perform an arabesque, she could not get the rotation or the elongation from the front of her trunk, so she compensated at the SI joint and pelvis, EVERY TIME. If you look at the photo, you can see this clearly.

The SI joint can be challenging at times because the common thinking is that "my SI joint goes out." What does that mean exactly? What goes out? Was there a pop or does it just hurt? In her case, the SI joint was the poor victim.

There is a school of thought that asserts that just because a person stands in a "weird" or "non-optimal" position, this does not necessarily result in pain.[91] I happen to agree.

Your posture is your own and many people have been standing the same way for years and are fine. For others, that non-optimal position results in pain. As I've said before, your situation is unique and should be evaluated as such.

What I Found

However, there are instances when standing or standing and moving your limbs is the chief complaint, which was the case here. Posture can be an important component of the evaluation, especially in the case of a dancer. It is the starting point for many movement patterns. When I performed a standing postural evaluation, the patient presented with a rotation in her pelvis to the left side. Simply put, the lower part of her torso was turned to the left. Not surprising.

Additionally, I found some restrictions in her trunk (thorax) that could possibly be compensatory. These compensations or adjustments from our nervous system help us in certain situations, until we run out of options. In her situation, because of the chronic overuse of her abdominal muscles, the compensation manifested as a tendency for her upper body to turn right.

When we see twists like this, we often consider the chicken or egg scenario. Was the pelvis rotated to the left because the upper body was rotated to the right, or vice versa? This is all well and good. Does it matter? Movement is the key. *We need to see what happens dynamically.*

---

91   Refshauge, Kathryn; Boist, Leonard; Goodsell, Michalene. "The Relationship Between Cervicothoracic Posture and the Presence of Pain." Journal of Manual & Manipulative Therapy, Vol 3, Iss 1, 21-24, Jul 2013.

As a practitioner, the original cause of the rotation did not matter so much to me. Why? Because when I evaluated her movement, I looked for areas that were not moving optimally and tried to discover where the breakdown was occurring. When I evaluated the movement of her arabesque, standing on her right leg, I found the following.

- hiking of her left hip (causing her to complain of that "jamming" in her left SI joint)

- this hike caused her rib cage to shift to the right.

Try this: Hike your left hip up—whether you are standing on your right toes or not, you will notice a shift to your right side.

At this point, the brain makes a decision by asking the following question: Do I compensate or do I let the person fall over to the right?

In her case the brain said, "I'll compensate for this."

The brain helped her compensate by shifting all her weight back onto her left side. Since her left leg was in the air, this had to happen via the left part of her trunk. This would be challenging for the average person, but since she was very flexible and a seasoned dancer, the shift was easy. In that way, all parts were in sync, so to speak—at least that's what her brain thought: *Now I can face forward!*

After evaluating her in the arabesque position, I tested her leg kick backwards while she was on her tummy in a much less loaded position. (I performed the same test on the other person with pelvic pain—see page 112). The same compensations presented themselves. Unfortunately, this all came with a price. Compensations always do. The price in her case happened to be a loss of control in her trunk (thorax) as well as the inability to control her movement without pain. I had found the cause of her pain.

As I have mentioned in other areas of the book, when I look at a movement—in her case, the arabesque—I look for areas that are not moving optimally. I play one area off of another until I find an area that, when modified, will restore almost normal movement (for that person) and leave them feeling little to no discomfort. When that is done, I hone in on the area that I believe to be the cause and then assess for muscle and joint restrictions.

The soft tissue restrictions I found here were of no surprise:

- External and internal oblique muscles

- Rectus abdominis

- Serratus anterior

- Diaphragm

These are all muscles of the trunk and I expected restrictions in this case, considering her story of the sustained positions she had to maintain during the opera performance. When we improved the control in her rib cage, she was able to perform the arabesque pain-free. Now the trick was to train her brain to do this!

What Worked

The ultimate goal of her treatment program was to replace her non-optimal strategy with a more efficient and effective one. She needed to develop a new habit, so to speak. Old habits are hard to break but with discipline and the right dose of training, it can be done.

What I did

- Soft tissue releases to the diaphragm and external and internal obliques, those muscles that had been causing compensations and were constantly overworked during her opera performance.

- Yoga poses—child's pose and down dog—to open up the thorax

- Taped the thorax to help with control[92] (see page 88 for photo)

- Trained movement and motor control in loaded and unloaded positions. Think no weight progressing to full-body weight challenges.

- Trained new motor patterns in the brain

Initially, I performed soft tissue releases with a combination of techniques to release certain muscles—the external and internal obliques and diaphragm—that were causing these compensations. Because of the way she had to sit for her opera performance, these particular muscles were extremely overworked and tugging on her rib cage. When they are overused, as was the case here, they caused a compensation in her thorax, thus preventing her from controlling the movement effectively.

I used child's pose and down dog to effectively open up the thorax. Taping to the ribcage was also used initially to help with the control. This was very helpful for her! When she took a dance class after one of our sessions (with the tape still on), a weakness in her hip became very apparent. She told me that she was standing at the barre on one leg and it was shaking! That's the game changer.

---

92   Lee, Diane and Lee, Linda Joy (LJ). *Discover Physio Series*, Vancouver, B.C., 2012.

When you take away a person's compensation, it will undoubtedly reveal a weakness or a restriction you did not know they had.

We then proceeded to train her movement and motor control, as well as spend time training her brain, as this was the heart of the problem. Remember, the brain is very smart and it will take the path of least resistance, so we need to train a new motor pattern in physical therapy. Practiced movement makes *permanent*, not perfect.

> **When you take away a person's compensation, it will undoubtedly reveal a weakness or a restriction you did not know they had.**

First, we did a series of movements in less challenging positions than her arabesque. We then progressed her to standing on one leg and eventually to a full arabesque. The neuro-muscular part and the brain training included repeated practice, so this can be ingrained as a movement pattern in her brain. Ever hear of neuroplasticity?[93] This is the concept at its best. Train the brain and the brain will adapt.

The mental cueing and imagery that worked for my patient was "Imagine you have space in your ribcage. Lengthen and align."[94]

She could perform a one-legged bridge, which provided for stability in the one-legged standing position. Next, we progressed to a standing position and having her kick her left leg back. The standing hip position is certainly more functional, and it directly relates to her arabesque position.

She was also a Pilates instructor. Because of that experience, we worked together to figure out exercises on the various Pilates equipment that supported her goals.

---

93   **Neuroplasticity** refers to the potential that the brain has to reorganize itself by creating new neural pathways to adapt, as it needs.

94   Franklin, Eric. Dance Imagery for Technique and Performance, 2nd edition. Human Kinetics: 2013.

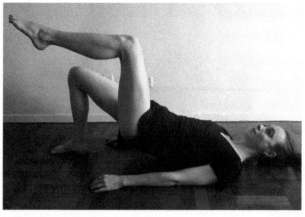

Single Leg Bridge

In her case, the primary source for left SI joint pain was in her thorax, so her treatment revolved around addressing the compensations in that area as well as correcting the movements she would need to perform in her daily routine.

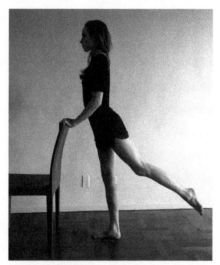

Standing Hip Extension

The treatment was exceptionally successful, and she was able to resume her demanding dance schedule, as well as her opera obligations, with increased strength and greater knowledge as to the prevention and management of her injury for the future.

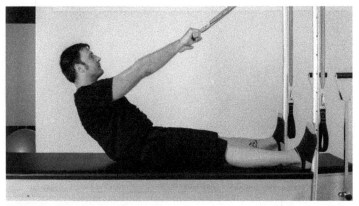

Pilates: seated roll downs to decompress the thorax

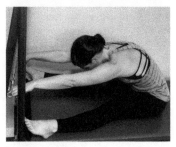

Seated push-throughs

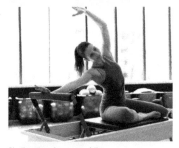

Challenging the arms while controlling the thorax

Positive Results

- Pain-free once she learned to control her movement in her thorax

- Increased strength in her hip muscles

- A new motor pattern in her brain

- An understanding of what to do with regards to prevention and management

Elite athletes
in pain have
uncontrolled
movement
patterns

Really? My **right** shoulder pain is due to an old shoulder issue on my **left side**?

Did you know that your shoulder pain can be caused by a restriction in your opposite shoulder? Or that it can be caused by a restriction in other joints surrounding the shoulder?

Truth

The shoulder is a ball-and-socket joint, much like the hip. Limitations could include the inability to move the arm in different planes of motion (i.e., overhead, behind the back, etc.). Other issues could include the inability to do a push-up, a pull-up or even a bench press. Reaching out in front of your body can even be difficult.

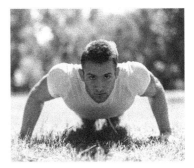

As you can see from this photo, a push-up puts a fair amount of stress on the shoulder. If there is more weight put on one arm during this movement, it can be difficult to execute efficiently.

Reaching your arm out in front of your body may be difficult if you have restrictions in your symptomatic shoulder. Sometimes it feels fine, sometimes it does not.

Imagine if you have restrictions on the other side.

Try this: Reach your right arm out in front of your body as if you were reaching for something on a shelf. Note the ease and amplitude of movement. Now turn your trunk to the right a little. Then repeat the reaching task, and you will notice a change.

Those subtle shifts do change the mechanics of the upper body, however subtle they may feel, especially if you have a shoulder issue. You may not even notice them until you start to load your shoulder in a push-up or pull-up, for example. Shifts in our body are normal; it's part of life and how we move. However, when we increase the load to our system as in a push up, how our body deals with this increased stress becomes important.

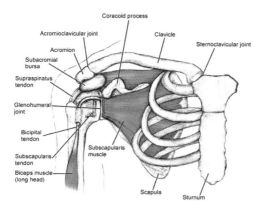

Our shoulder girdle is composed of many joints and muscles. As you can see from the photo at left, aside from the shoulder, we have the sternum, the rib cage, the collarbone (clavicle), as well as the scapula and the neck (not shown). As previously mentioned, the shoulder is a ball-and-socket joint and affords movement in multiple planes.

A limitation or increased mobility of any given joint could, by the nature of these anatomic relationships, affect the mobility or lack thereof in the shoulder joint itself. When you present with shoulder pain, a physician may give you a diagnosis of bursitis, tendonitis, or shoulder impingement,[95] but WHAT is causing you to have this condition or problem?

The shoulder can ultimately be the victim, but as always we want to find out where the *primary source* of the problem lies. It may be in the shoulder, or it may not. My experience has shown me that with chronic

---

95   A shoulder impingement is a clinical syndrome where the tendons of the rotator cuff muscles become irritated and inflamed as they pass through the subacromial space, the passage beneath the acromion. This can result in pain, weakness, and loss of movement at the shoulder.

shoulder problems, there is often another area of the body that is involved. Sometimes it's the neck, often it is the shoulder blade (scapula), or it can also come from the upper rib cage. You may have a stiff joint, a nerve injury, a muscle imbalance, or even an abdominal restriction that limits overhead movement. Your nervous system chooses which strategy works best depending on the movement.

The shoulder pain can also come from your other side, as it did in these two people.

Story

Two of my patients were very active, and in great shape, but neither one of them was able to do a series of push-ups without shoulder pain. The first person (Person 1) had a history of shoulder surgery on his opposite shoulder, and the second person (Person 2) had significant scar tissue from a previous injury, also on his opposite side. In addition, when Person 1 did a bench press, he told me that he always rotated to the right, making his left arm higher than his right.

Both complained of shoulder pain that worsened with the movements described above. Person 1 had a history of multiple injuries and a surgery to repair the labrum[96] in his left shoulder some years back.

Person 2 had sustained a fracture of his left collarbone, some years back as well.

One had physical therapy elsewhere with little relief, and the other had been receiving repeated cortisone injections to the shoulder by a physician in NYC and was given a diagnosis of AC (acromial-clavicular) arthritis, also with not much relief. Yes, he probably had some degenerative changes in his AC joint, but that was not the cause of this problem.

Both had high goals when it came to their fitness, and if they could not perform a bench press or even a push-up without pain, it would have a significant effect on their performance goals. Everyone is different when it comes to their fitness goals. However, when I have two individuals who are in excellent

---

96   The labrum in the shoulder is defined as a ring of fibrocartiliage that runs around the cavity of the scapula (shoulder blade) in which the head of the humerus (upper arm bone) fits.

physical shape come to me with complaints of shoulder pain, then a goal of just reaching over their head without pain is not good enough.

To begin their evaluations, I looked at how each one of them performed a push-up or a bench press to start. If you have shoulder pain with a bench press, and if that is the only time it occurs, then it is obvious that your bench press must be evaluated. If that kind of focused evaluation is not happening, then you should ask your health care provider to do it. Evaluation of the movement that causes you problems is integral to your understanding and recovery.

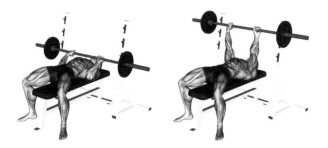

Most people are so concerned with getting the weight off their chest and pushing the bar up, that at times their form is compromised. Often, the problem lies in the weight being too heavy.

However, as we've learned about compensations, you can bet that if the body can compensate and push that weight up, it will. The body will use accessory muscles to complete the movement. If you are hypermobile[97] like Person 1, you will be able to push past your end range of motion repeatedly and possibly give yourself an arthritic joint.[98] Do that often enough, and you run the risk of an overuse injury.

Good physical therapists are experts at analyzing and restoring optimal movement. We look for buckle points in these movement patterns that may be contributing to the problem.

---

97   Hypermobile means that you have joints that move beyond the normal range of motion. Put more simply, think very flexible.

98   Beighton, PH; Grahame, R. Hypermobility of Joints, 3rd ed. London: Springer-Veriag, 1999.

What I Found

In the initial evaluation for Person 1, I found a restriction in his upper ribs (thorax) on the side that had the shoulder surgery (left). This caused a compensatory rotation to the right side in his upper body.

In order to get the right arm down to the ground at the same time as the left when he performed a push-up, he had to push further with his right side. This extra push on the right side ultimately increased the wear and tear on that side, which resulted in the beginnings of a somewhat arthritic shoulder. The same thing happened with the bench press.

Try this: Rotate your upper body to the right with your arms outstretched in front of your body. You will see that the right arm is farther back than the left, thus increasing the distance that the arm has to move when performing movement out in front of your body.

Other pertinent issues with this patient included:

- Soft tissue restrictions on his left side, which included serratus anterior, pectoralis minor, and intercostal muscles

- These muscles were gripping and causing him to lose control in his upper body when he did a push-up, for example. As you can see from the photo on page 48, they attach to the ribs; when they are overworked, they can add to the dysfunction in the area.

- A lack of rotational control with his right shoulder when performing exercises with heavy weight

- Limited mobility in his left shoulder

In the initial evaluation of Person 2, we found similar issues, plus a secondary issue with the shoulder blade on the same side of his shoulder pain.

- A restriction in the upper chest from an old collarbone fracture on his left side

- Increased tone in his right rhomboids and levator scapula muscles

- These, in turn, positioned the scapula (shoulder blade) in a non-optimal position

What Worked

Both patients presented with the same symptom, but we were able to prescribe custom treatment regimens that included taping, soft tissue release, and manual therapy techniques when needed. They did indeed present with similar symptoms, but the cause of their problem was a bit different.

What I did

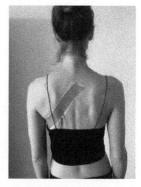

- Taping to their upper ribs on the opposite side as well as taping to unload the shoulder blade for Person 2. (See page 56 for photos of upper rib taping and see photo to the right for the shoulder blade (scapula) taping.)

- Soft tissue release for the muscles that were preventing the upper ribs from moving effectively as well as soft tissue work on the shoulder blade.

The taping produced an immediate decrease in the overall pain level and increased the ability to perform a push-up. However, tape is not a permanent fix, so the muscles and movement patterns needed to be retrained.

Retraining the muscles and movement patterns is the key to permanent change for many people. Increasing awareness and educating these patients as to source of the problem also enables them to understand what to do to maintain the gains made in physical therapy as well as to prevent the issue from happening again in the future.

Since their impairment was rotation, and rotational control, a series of corrective exercises to achieve this control was necessary. We could start them lying on their back performing triceps extensions. This trains load in a short lever movement, which differs from a full push-up featuring a longer lever as the arms go from fully straight to fully bent.

Another option is to start them on their back with knees bent and introduce exercises with weights (pictured at right).

Corrective exercise could then progress to a series of push-ups against the wall with rotation introduced accordingly.

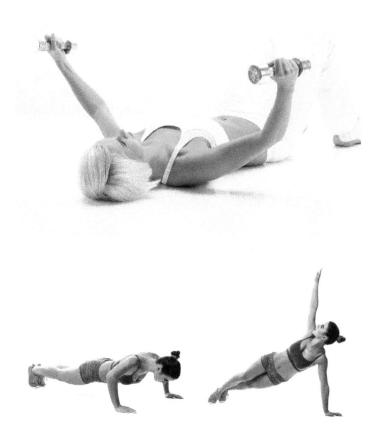

Another corrective exercise may include a full plank against the wall with rotation to one side and eventual progression to the floor (as above).

These exercises all train CONTROL. Both of these patients were already fairly strong, so just plain vanilla cookie cutter rotator cuff or upper body strengthening would NEVER make them better. Right?

What they lacked was the *control* to push a bar up or do a full body weight push-up. When the biomechanics of the movement were corrected, and their nervous system adjusted to this new movement pattern, it was apparent that the power and skill that they thought they had was not there. *You take away someone's compensation, and the reality unfolds.*

Another movement practice could include a triangle pose in yoga to open up the upper rib cage. If Pilates equipment is available, one could do seated roll-downs with rotation on the Cadillac (see page 147 for picture).

This exercise is done to train an optimal strategy for movement and retrain a new motor map in the brain. Remember: "Practice makes permanent, not perfect." These exercises and movements must be done repeatedly so they can be patterned, almost like a new habit.[99]

"You take away someone's compensation, and the reality unfolds."

How movement is controlled is vital. It is not just about the quantity of movements, push-ups, or bench presses in this case; it is about the quality of the movement and how these patients can coordinate other muscles and joints in an effective and beautiful move.

These are just samples of corrective exercises and movement retraining. There are many other types of exercises you can do, but that is beyond the scope of this book. The one important takeaway here is that the retraining must be SPECIFIC to the patient. One size DOES NOT fit all in this scenario or in the other stories in this book.

Positive Results

- The ability to do a push-up and bench press without pain!

- Given their active status, they can now progress their weight-training program and work with their personal trainer to achieve peak performance!

- The knowledge of what to do in case they fall back into their faulty patterns in the future.

---

99   Shumway-Cook, Ann. Motor Control: Translating Research into Clinical Practice, 4th edition. LWW: 2011.

lengthen
align
strengthen

Chapter 10

Really? My **shoulder** has not improved because my **neck** is stiff?

Did you know that the inability to lift your arm up or put your hand behind your back may be due to a restriction in your neck? Not all shoulder problems stem from a problem in the shoulder, especially if the problem is a chronic one.

Truth

The shoulder and the neck are so closely related anatomically that synchronous movement happens when all those structures work effectively together. Take the hand behind the back, for example.

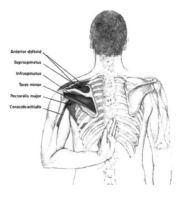

As you see from the picture on the next page, there are many connections between the muscles and joints of the shoulder and the upper neck. I have many a patient who has compensated with their neck when they are unable to reach up and scratch their back or put on their bra.

Is your shoulder pain really a neck problem?[100]

_____

100   Smebrano, Jonathan N; Yson, Sharon C; Kanu, Okezika C; Braman, Jonathan P; Santos, Edward Rainer G; Harrison, Alicia K; Polly, David W. Jr. "Neck-Shoulder Crossover: How Often Do Neck and Shoulder Pathology Masquerade as Each Other?" Journal of Orthopedics, Vol 42, Iss 9, 76-80, Sept 2013.

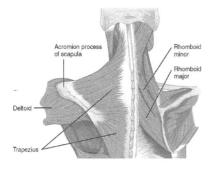

Acromion process
of scapula

Rhomboid
minor

Rhomboid
major

Deltoid

Trapezius

I have personal experience with this type of restriction since I have a very tight upper neck. I sustained an injury about two years ago to my right shoulder, and one of the major restrictions was an inability to move my arm back and also an inability to put my hand behind my back and reach up. This chronic neck issue occasionally restricts dynamic motions of both of my arms as well. However, when I am able to release these muscles manually or from a stretch, I am able to extend my hand up much higher. Every time I reached my hand behind my back, I felt a pull in my upper neck. When that pull was released—or taken away, so to speak—I could reach up much further.

Another example of a shoulder movement restriction can originate when lifting your arm up as if you are following through on a throwing motion. Your arm is out to the side and you are reaching forward or down, similar to a baseball pitch. See below.

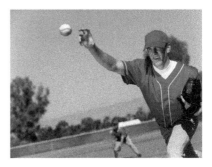

This is a very common problem in people with shoulder pain. Since it is a ball-and-socket joint, it functions in three planes, or "3D," as I like to call it. If you have problems lifting your arm out to the side combined with another motion, usually rotation, then all sorts of compensations start to abound, especially in throwing athletes because they need to use these combined motions as part of an effective throwing motion.

If your neck is playing into the problem, there will be a greater ease of movement when you change its position.

I am mentioning this only because your neck needs to be assessed when you have a shoulder problem. This may seem basic, but more often than not, these issues are missed because a full assessment of the neck and shoulder girdle is not done. Remember, dynamic movement requires mobility and control at multiple joints.[101]

Story

A woman came to see me with complaints of right shoulder pain. She was unable to put her hand behind her back or lift up her arm as if to hail a taxi. We are in NYC, after all! She had physical therapy in another country, where she was from, which was focused on strengthening.

I believe that if you strengthen muscles that are playing into faulty or non-optimal biomechanics, then you strengthen for nothing. Why? Because you are only as strong as your range of motion allows. Not to mention the fact that you are reinforcing a poor movement pattern.

For example, if you can lift your arm up halfway and can do it fairly well, that's great. But what about the rest of the range? If you cannot lift your arm up all the way, then all the strengthening in the world won't get your arm up further if the REASON why you do not have full range is not addressed.

The body does not operate in isolated segments, but it functions as a dynamic unit enabling us to use familiar movement patterns, even with such a simple movement as lifting your arm up. That is why it is so important to integrate these movements as part of the clinical assessment.

This was the case in this person's story. She came in with complaints of right shoulder pain. The two main problems were her inability to put her hand behind her back as well as to lift her arm up to the side with her elbow flexed (bent). See photo on prior page, similar to baseball throw position.

A hot shower and a massage were the only things that made her feel better. At times, she had difficulty sleeping on that side as well, which is common in people who have shoulder issues.

---

101   Chu, Samuel K; Jayabalan, Prakash; Kibler, W. Ben; Press, Joel. "The Kinetic Chain Revisited: New Concepts on Throwing Mechanics and Injury." Physical Medicine & Rehab, Vol 8, Iss 3, S69-S77, Mar 2016.

What I Found

On initial assessment, her right shoulder appeared forward and anterior, which also is not unusual for a right-hand dominant individual, especially if you use that hand for most of your daily activities. As a matter of fact, her entire shoulder girdle was rotated to the left.

I took a look at the two movements that were important to her during the assessment. When she put her hand behind her back, her right shoulder elevated, her neck shifted to the right and her symptoms were reproduced. Those are not normal mechanics when you move your hand in that way. Either these were compensations for something happening in the shoulder, or they were the true cause of the problem. Ultimately, that was her strategy. Her nervous system decided to perform the movement in that way. It works for awhile, until you run out of options.

If you take a look at the anatomy of the neck and its relationship to the shoulder from the images on the preceding pages, you can see that if there is a pull from above in the neck, or vice-versa, it will hinder or help movement of the arm depending on the movement.

If you are a visual learner like myself, you can imagine how if there is a pull from one muscle in the neck, that tension may alter the inter-relationships of the surrounding musculature.

Furthermore, as we get older and develop degenerative conditions in the neck, they may—by virtue of the aging process—cause compensations in other parts of the neck and shoulder complex.

Tightness in the muscles in our upper neck can alter the mechanics of the neck, shoulder girdle, and upper rib cage. This compensation is also quite common because many people adopt that typical "leaning forward" posture to look at their computer screens, tablets, etc.

Additionally, when she placed her hand behind her back, her shoulder tipped forward excessively as well, but that came later in the motion. With a combined movement like this, things generally go wrong at the beginning of the movement. In the end, changing the position of her neck enabled her to reach up behind her back easier and farther.

I then looked at the other movement that bothered her, taking her arm up to the side with her elbow flexed and her forearm down—similar to part of the baseball throw mentioned previously in the story.

I saw the same issue with the neck, but I also saw her shoulder and her upper body turn to the left, which is also not typical for that motion. Improving the neck position also made this movement better and decreased her symptoms. Her shoulder girdle still was not optimal, albeit to a lesser extent.

When I changed the position of her shoulder manually, which was not easy to do, she was better able to move the arm as well. With all these modifications, I was giving her nervous system another option to move.

What Worked

Since I believed the neck to be the prime cause of both of her problems, I started there. In my initial assessment, I determined that the mobility in the upper part of her neck was restricted and thereby changed how she moved her neck as well as her arm.

What I did

- Soft tissue release to upper neck muscles

- Manual therapy to upper neck

- Chin tucks on foam roller (see photo of chin tucks on page 146)

- Standing chin tuck with addition of hand movement behind back

- Muscle releases to upper rib cage (intercostal muscles, serratus anterior muscles, and pec major and minor muscles; see page 48 for images)

- Corrective exercises to increase the movement of her right arm as she raised it above her shoulder

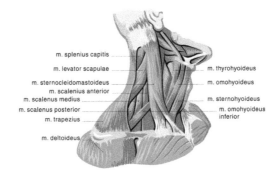

I performed some soft tissue release to the muscles in her upper neck. As you can see in the picture above, there are many layers to the muscles of the neck. They are not large muscles but can perpetuate a headache as well as an upper extremity problem. These also become restricted in a typical forward head posture.

I also implemented some manual therapy to her upper neck as well—not because she had a stiff joint, but to dampen down the tone in these muscles.[102]

Ultimately, with all these treatment strategies, we are trying to affect the nervous system in a positive way. This is explained in other sections in the book, but people who are in persistent pain generally have a sensitized nervous system and, simply put, the goal is to decrease this sensitivity with the many tools we have in our toolboxes.[103]

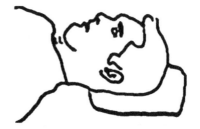

She also performed chin tucks on a foam roll (if you don't have a foam roll, you can do this exercise on the ground with a towel) to lengthen her upper neck. She then added some neck rotation to the movement.

I then had her progress to performing this movement in a standing position while she put her hand behind her back. This is certainly practical, if not functional!

The patient also did Pilates, so we incorporated this into her routine. More specifically, on the Cadillac using the bar, she sat back with her right arm out to the side while keeping her upper neck lengthened. See next page for a visual on this.

---

102   Clinical Experience

103   Butler, David. The Sensitive Nervous System, 1st Edition. OPTP: 2006.

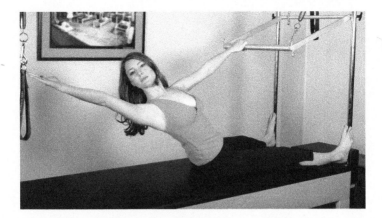

With the movement of the hand behind the back addressed, we then moved on to treating the other motion that bothered her—taking her arm out to the side. The neck work helped her a lot, but it did not enable her to lift her arm up all the way.

When I manually corrected the position of her shoulder in the evaluation, I felt that certain muscles were prohibiting her shoulder from moving well. Based on that assessment, I performed releases to the muscles of her upper rib cage (intercostal muscles, serratus anterior, as well as her pec major and minor). This was done via breath work, MET (muscle energy technique),[104] as well as traditional release techniques. These are also described in other sections of the book, as they are common muscles that tend to inhibit movement in our upper extremity.

I wanted to change her strategy for not only moving her hand behind her back but also lifting it up and out to the side. To that end, this movement strategy is akin to changing a habit—and habits are hard to break unless you really work at them! This strategy implementation requires more than just mindless practice; it requires mindful movement and focus.

---

104   Chaitow, Leon. Muscle Energy Techniques, 4th Edition. Churchill Livingstone: 2013.

Some of her practices included the child's pose (below).

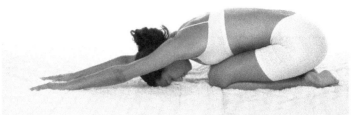

This was done to lengthen her rib cage (thorax). Remember, the intercostal muscles and serratus anterior attach there. You could also incorporate the chin tuck with movement to further lengthen the neck.

She also did a traditional thoracic opener technique. I had her do this to the right, because that is where her restriction was. A lot of people ask me, "Should I do both sides?" the answer to that question depends on what you are doing. In this patient's case, her path of least resistance was to the left, which was seen during the initial assessment. So why would I want to reinforce a faulty movement pattern by doing both sides? The brain would get really confused!

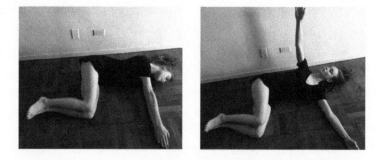

These were the mainstays of her program. Sometimes less is more. You do not have to do a million different exercises just to get your hand behind your back or to move your arm up and out to the side. Each plan is geared toward the individual, which means her treatment was specific to her.

Sometimes the brain responds to different exercises put in the program at different times. This is certainly true and depends on the chronicity of the problem.[105]

Results

The patient responded well to this treatment program and was able to move her arm freely in all planes of motion. Since she was not overloaded with exercises, she was able to incorporate these into her Pilates program as well as her weekly routine. In this way, the new strategies and movements we introduced during treatment became grounded in her daily system, eventually turned into habits, and became effective tools for prevention as well.

Remember, if your shoulder problem is not getting better, consider another source to the problem. It could be your neck, or it could be something else. Advocate for yourself and have your practitioner do some detective work.

105   Carlino, E.; Benedetti, F. "Different contexts, different pains, different experiences." Neuroscience. Elsevier, Ltd.: Dec 2016.

Your **life** is worth **more** than a bottle of pills

Chapter 11

Really? The source of my **knee** pain comes from my **hip** and **foot**?

Did you know that if you have problems kneeling, the cause could potentially be in your hip or even your foot?

Truth

As I mentioned in the other story on the knee (competitive golfer with knee pain), the knee is often the victim in most cases. If you don't look above and below the knee, the source of the problem could easily be missed.

As you can see from the photo, kneeling requires the synergistic action from both your hips and feet, let alone the ability to stand up from this posture, which requires good hip and knee strength.

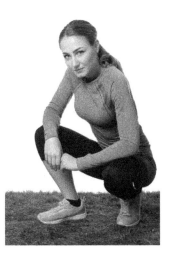

The ability to maintain this posture is another story. When you are kneeling in this position, your knee joint is at its end range of motion,[106] not to mention the fact that you have a percentage of your body weight testing this range as well.

---

106   Range of motion is defined as the measurement of movement around a joint.

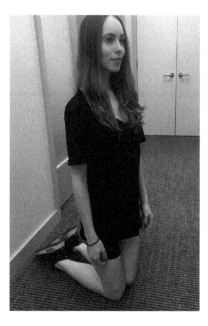

Your quadriceps muscles are on a bit of a stretch, and your hips are in a flexed (bent) position. You could be kneeling turned to one side or kneeling straight ahead. Contrast that with the more neutral hip position you see here with kneeling at ninety degrees.

Kneeling at ninety degrees of knee flexion,[107] versus kneeling at full flexion, will result in varying forces across the knee joint.[108] However, if you have knee pain when your knee is bent all the way, then kneeling like the person in the first picture may be problematic, which was the case with my patient.

We do not realize that we have to kneel a lot in our daily activities— reaching for something on a bottom shelf or kneeling down to play with your children on the floor, for example. I once had a patient who was a pre-school teacher and the amount of time she had to kneel on the floor on any given day was mind boggling! Even in my own practice, I kneel quite often!

Story

A thirty-five-year-old female was referred to me with complains of left knee pain "behind my knee," as she put it, or in the region that is between the back of the thigh and the calf. In my language, we call it the *popliteal fossa*.

She felt it most while kneeling playing with her child on the floor as well as while crossing her legs. She also felt it after running. She had a previous history of knee pain about two years prior that resolved on its own, she then gave birth to a baby girl who was a little over a year old at the time

---

107   Flexion: think "bending the knee"

108   Pollard, Jonisha P.; Porter, William L.; Redfern, Mark S. "Forces and Moments on the Knee During Kneeling and Squatting." Journal of Applied Biomechanics. 2011 Aug 27 (3): 233-41.

of the initial evaluation. It is well-known that throughout pregnancy, ligaments increase their laxity and the body undergoes a series of biomechanical, hormonal, and vascular changes that can result in a variety of musculoskeletal disorders.[109]

There have also been reports of maternal peripheral nerve injuries during labor and delivery, affecting both the sensory and motor nerves.[110] This not only affects sensation, but strength as well.

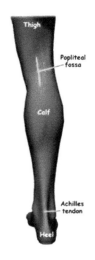

She was fairly active and enjoyed running, Pilates, working out on the elliptical, and the occasional Barre class. The patient expressed that her knee pain was always worse at the end of the day. She shared that she carried her baby on her right hip, which I knew altered the weight bearing position of her left leg. She had no X-rays or any other imaging when she was referred to me by her husband, whom I had treated on prior occasions.

Performing a differential diagnosis, you could make a case for hormonal changes during pregnancy and thereafter affecting the quality of her ligaments. She was also a bit too young to have osteoarthritis and had no problems walking. She did not meet any of the criteria for fibromyalgia, rheumatoid arthritis, and a host of other potential inflammatory or non-inflammatory causes of knee pain. Additionally, she had no cognitive or emotional barriers that would impede or slow down her recovery. Consequently, I believed it to be mechanical with a small component of postpartum ligamentous laxity.

109   Proisy, Maia; Rouill, Alban; Raolt, Helene; Rozel, Celine; Guggenbuhl, Pascal; Jacob, Denis; Guilin, Raphael. "Imaging of Muscoluskeletal Disorders Related to Pregnancy." American Journal of Roentgenology, Musculoskeletal Review, Vol 202, Iss 4: Apr 2014.

110   Madson, Timothy James. "Functional Lower Extremity Deficits with Sensory Changes and Quadriceps Weakness in a 29-Year-Old Female Postlabor and Delivery." Journal of Women's Health Physical Therapy, Vol 38, Iss 1, 11-18, Apr 2014.

What I Found

Since she had a problem with "deep knee bends," I took a look at her squat (both single and double leg) as well as her position on the floor when she played with her daughter.

I always like to do a postural scan to determine a patient's baseline. Without getting into detail, of note was the left hip, which was more forward (anterior) than the right and rotated medially (think turned "in"). Her rear foot displayed more of a pronated or internally rotated position. This is how she presented and had functioned fine this way for two years since her last injury. (see photos below). So what is the issue now?

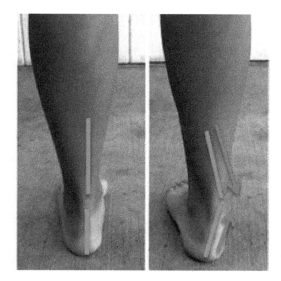

Additionally, she had knee symptoms when I had her bend her knee while lying on the table. As I mentioned in other sections in this book, our nervous system adapts to these new positions or strategies until one day, we reach our limit.

So now that I knew her starting point, I could assess what happened when she squatted (both single leg and double). Remember that running is a single leg activity. When I evaluated her squat on one leg, she continued to rotate her torso to the right (non-optimal), and her left knee also displayed abnormal movement. Above all, she still displayed poor mechanics at her feet as well. Her hip remained unchanged. As you can see from this photo, a one-legged squat is somewhat similar to the running form and therefore was a great starting point in the assessment.

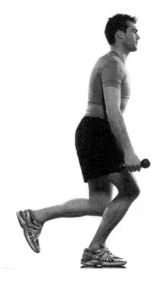

I then looked at how she side sat on her knees with her daughter. She sat with her RIGHT hip forward, not her left. She also had left knee pain in this position. We always have default or comfortable positions we sit in; it's called our path of least resistance! This caused her to put more weight onto her left thigh, which was already at its end range.

Exercise: You can try it—sit on the floor with both knees fully bent and your weight on your butt. Play with the rotation of your hips and see how it affects other parts of your body.

Adjusting her position in her squat by way of neutralizing the left foot provided the most relief for her with that movement. Additionally, when I modified her right hip position while she sat on the floor, she felt immediate relief in her knee. So at this point, I determined that treating her foot would help her running, and treating her hip will help her sit on the floor and enjoy the company of her daughter. Ultimately, we are giving you different options for movement.

Running and sitting on the floor are COMPLETELY different activities; one is loaded and the other is not. That is why your practitioner should look at *all* the activities that bother you—and not just one. You could have different sources to your problem, as this patient did. If I had only treated her foot, then sitting on the floor would still be a problem, and vice versa.

What Worked

Based on my assessment, I created a plan to address her needs.

What I did for her foot:

- Manual therapy to her foot

- Soft tissue (muscle) release to calf and foot intrinsic muscles

- Taping of midfoot for support and to optimize knee while running (see photo next page)

- Calf stretch on half foam roller (see page 114 for photo)

What I did for her hip:

- Soft tissue releases to the front hip muscles: *psoas* and *rectus femoris*

- Manual therapy with a mobilizing belt to increase hip flexion

- Quad stretch off the table

- Exercises on all fours to self-mobilize the right hip

As noted above, I treated her foot with a combination of manual therapy to her midfoot as well as soft tissue release to the muscles that were holding her foot in its non-optimal position. These muscles included the calf and some of the muscles at the bottom of her foot. We call these muscles the *intrinsics*.

When these muscles become hyperactive, they tend to act as a compressive force on the foot. It is important to note that many people walk around all day with these issues in their feet and have no problem. This patient had no problem walking either. But it was a factor in her running.

In order to better support her midfoot, I applied tape to lift or sling it. I used Leukotape (not Kinesio Tape—that is too stretchy for this application) with an undercover of Hypofix. Again, this supported her midfoot so she could optimize her knee mechanics while running.

After that, I checked her squat to reassess, and it was fine. I also sent her home the first day with a calf stretch on a half foam roller.

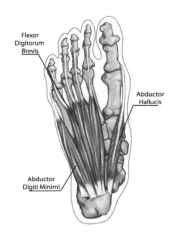

Flexor
Digitorum
Brevis

Abductor
Hallucis

Abductor
Digiti Minimi

Intrinsics

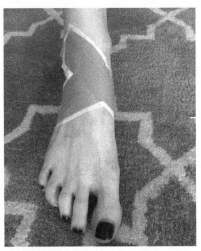

Midfoot taping - Navicular Lift

I then moved on to address her activity of kneeling on the floor. When I assessed the hip, I found certain muscles that were pulling her hip forward. Her hip joint was not stiff, per se, but some motions, especially flexion (think knee to chest), were restricted versus the other side. I felt this was relevant considering she needed a lot of hip flexion to sit on the floor in that position.

Treatment consisted of soft tissue releases to the muscles of the front of her hip (*psoas* and *rectus femoris*) and joint mobilizations with a belt to increase hip flexion.[111]

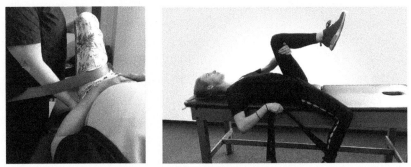

Hip mobilzation

Quad stretch off table

111   Mulligan, Brian R. Manual Therapy: Nags, Snags, MWMs, etc., 4th edition. Orthopedic Physical Therapy Products: 2010.

I also gave her a quadriceps stretch off the table as well as an exercise on all fours designed to self-mobilize the right hip (see page 79 for all fours exercise). She got down on all fours with her right hip in external rotation (think turned out), and then she rocked back about 75 percent. This helped seat her hip in its most optimal position.[112]

Positive Results

She was able to run and take her classes pain-free and, most of all, she was able to sit down on the floor and play with her child! Of note here, is that we treated her left foot and the *right* hip to help alleviate her left knee pain. As I've mentioned in the other stories, you will get better results if you are open to sources of your problem that lie beyond your symptomatic areas, especially if you have persistent, unsolved issues.

> "Celebrate your individuality with a treatment plan specifically geared toward your issues. "

Everybody is different as to how they react to such forces wherever they are applied, and these individual reactions are what make each of us unique. That is why there cannot be a "cookbook" approach applied to your rehab. What bothers someone else may not bother you. Celebrate your individuality with a treatment plan specifically geared toward *your* issues.

As stated previously, having this kind of global, comprehensive approach to rehab is absolutely crucial to long-term rehab success, and that's what you want, right? That's why you owe it to yourself to see a physical therapist who will honor your individuality with a whole-body clinical reasoning process and a treatment plan designed with your unique issues in mind.

---

112   Sahrmann, Shirley. Diagnosis and Treatment of Movement Impairment Syndromes, 1st ed. Mosby: 2001.

Practice like
a **champion**—
it makes
permanent,
not perfect

Really? My **knee** pain is not improving because of tightness in my **low-back**?

Did you know that your right knee pain could be a result of tightness on the left side of your trunk? Put simply, the inability to power through your golf swing could be related to the fact that you cannot weight shift from right to left due to a restriction on the left side of your body.

Truth

The golf swing is the epitome of the kinetic chain in all its beauty, and it incorporates pretty much every joint in your body.[113] The feet are generally fixed on the ground throughout the duration of the golf swing, although they obviously have some rotation due to the weight shift involved.

Having all of those joints involved is bound to introduce some compensations into the golf swing. If, for example, you have limited rotation in your hips, you could compensate in your low-back during the backswing or the follow-through.[114] This is actually very common. Something else to consider during your golf swing is that you might have a lot of movement in your hips, thereby over-rotating and also causing problems.

---

113   Chu, Yungchien; Sell, Timothy C; Lephart, Scott M. "The Relationship Between Biomechanical Variables and Driving Performance During the Golf Swing." Sports Sciences, Vol 28, 1251-59, Sept 2010.

114   Kim, Sol-Bi; You, Joshua (Sung) H; Kwon, Oh-Yun; Yi, Chung-Yi. "Lumbopelvic Kinematic Characteristics of Golfers with Limited Hip Rotation." American Journal of Sports Medicine, Sept 2014.

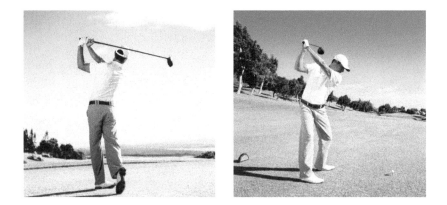

For the stiff hips, lack of mobility is the problem. For the mobile hips, lack of control is the issue. Both scenarios may have back pain and similar symptoms, but their treatment is certainly going to be vastly different.

With knee pain, you could have a similar scenario. For the right-handed golfer, you may over-twist your right knee on the downswing because you cannot control your pelvis. How come?

Some possible causes:

- Stiffness on the left side of your abdomen and back

- Restriction in your right or left foot (preventing them from pronating or supinating), thereby causing the knee to take the rotation

- Inability to turn your head to the left and having to rotate down the kinetic chain

- Improper weight shift

Similar symptoms, different causes. These are just a few possibilities.

Whatever it is, this all impacts your center of mass. It is this sense of body center that will impact the ground reaction force through your legs and will affect your ability to drive the ball.

When we ask our body to do a task that involves multiple movements at different joints, we better be sure that all these joints are in sync with one another, or eventually a breakdown will occur. If you are hypermobile, this breakdown may happen later on because you can easily adapt and compensate elsewhere, as your nervous system is highly adaptable. It is this lack of muscular control that is so crucial to identify and correct.[115]

That is why it is so important to have an integrated body assessment by a good physiotherapist. This is important for every patient, but with the golfer, there are so many dynamic movement patterns at work that it is absolutely vital to break these down to see where the dysfunction lies. Notice I did not say *pain*, but I said *dysfunction*.

As a golfer, you want to release any barriers that are interfering with both your short and long game and bolster your overall sport performance.

Story

A competitive golfer came to me with longstanding complaints of right knee pain. Prior to this, he had been seen by a few physicians and physical therapists as well. He played through the pain, but by the end of a round of golf, he was really sore. He wore a knee brace, but that does not protect the knee if another part of the body is the source of the pain in the first place. His knee pain came on at a specific point in the golf swing—the downswing.

He had been told that he had weak quads and that he should "strengthen his knees" and increase his hamstring and glute strength. Certainly, he got stronger, but his knee pain persisted. To say the least, this would be a frustrating scenario for anyone, let alone a competitive athlete. As an aside, he had a history of concussion.

Due to the significant weight shift and force involved in the golf swing, the knee is the one joint that really gets stuck in the middle, between the hips that are rotating like crazy and the feet that are initiating the weight shift.

Although this is a chip shot sequence, you can see from the picture on the next page that when you drop your pelvis down to the right (fourth and fifth images on the right), there is an increased torque at the knee. This is normal. However, when you start to overcompensate at the pelvis because

---

115   Corkery, Marie B; O'Rourke, Brittany; Viola, Samantha; Sheng-Che, Yen; Rigby, Joseph. "An Exploratory Examination of the Association Between Altered Lumbar Motor Control, Joint Mobility and Low-back Pain in Athletes. Asian Journal of Sports Medicine, Vol 5, Iss 4, Dec 2014.

of an insufficient weight transfer, that is when you have to question, "Why is this happening?"

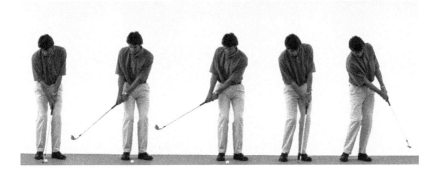

You could do that over and over again for months, offsetting the movement at other joints, until one day you can't compensate anymore. In addition to the knee pain with the downswing, he also said he had problems squatting and going up and down stairs.

" When you have a scenario like this, you have to break the cycle with rehab, movement, and brain training. "

Once you develop a faulty motor pattern, it carries over to other activities as well, especially since both squatting and stairs require increased activity at the knee and its surrounding muscles. Over time, especially if the problem is chronic, the body will take the path of least resistance. If you do the same thing over and over—dropping the pelvis, rotating your knee, and not weight shifting properly—the body and brain will think that is normal movement and will eventually adapt.

It is like a vicious cycle. When you have a scenario like this, you have to break the cycle with rehab, movement, and brain training. The pattern is so ingrained in your brain that you have to work extremely hard to develop a new strategy to create a new norm.

This includes varying the context in which you train as well as what types of training you do. As a matter of fact, it has been shown in research that the effects of synchronized time training via a metronome, for example, has a positive influence on neurophysiological motor programs and skill performance in golfers.[116]

Think of the simple analogy of an ankle injury, for example. You limp for a while, the pain eventually goes away, yet you are still limping. You have no more pain, but the limping is a habit you adopted after the initial injury to offload your painful ankle.

What I Found

This golfer's overall postural assessment revealed that just in standing he was bearing a lot of weight on his right leg. This is not the most optimal starting position for golf. You have to work really hard in this position to get all the weight over to the left through the swing.

You would think that it would be the opposite since it was his right knee that hurt. However, as I mentioned above, when you develop these patterns, they become your norm—not just in golf but in everyday life, like simply standing still.

When I tried to shift his weight to the left, his hip and pelvis dropped to the right. I then tried to stabilize the pelvis manually and weight shift him myself. I could only go so far, and then the force from the pelvis was so strong that the pelvis had to drop and his knee began to hurt. I had found the underlying compensation and ultimately the cause of his knee pain.

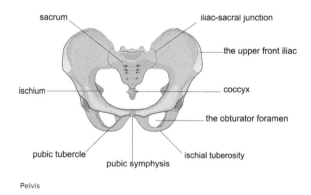

Pelvis

---

116   Sommer, Marius. "Effect of Time Training in Golf and Soccer Players." Doctoral thesis: Umea University, Faculty of Social Sciences, Department of Psychology, 2014.

I asked him what he felt when I tried to control his pelvis, and he told me that he felt a pull on the left side of his abdomen and his low-back.

Even in the basic standing position, a restriction or tightness on one side of the body can result in some form of compensation and may eventually cause hip or knee pain, for example.

You don't have to be a golfer to experience this. Imagine you are in a standing job all day, where you shift your weight from one side to the other. However, imagine doing that all day long for five days a week. If you do have a restriction like this person, it may manifest into something else. It may not. I only mention this as people do not realize that what they do all day long can be one of the contributing factors to their pain presentation. I know that while I am standing for a long period, I tend to place most of my weight on my right leg.

Since the downswing was the point in the golf swing where the patient had knee pain, that's where I eventually progressed in the evaluation. For starters, I evaluated his trunk rotation, first in sitting. This was normal, actually *more* than normal. If you are a golfer seeing a physical therapist, please make sure your rotation is evaluated no matter where your symptoms are presenting.[117]

" People do not realize that what they do all day long can be one of the contributing factors to their pain presentation. "

I concluded from this part of the evaluation that lack of rotation was certainly not the issue. For golfers at least, if you can't rotate from your thoracic spine (mid-back) in sitting, that's a problem. You can be checked in a standing position, but make sure someone stabilizes your hips so that pure rotation can be checked. It is too easy to compensate at the hips with this one. Obviously, you need hip rotation for golf, but your thorax must rotate or you will over-rotate somewhere else.[118]

---

117   Lindsay, David M., Horton, John F. "Trunk Rotation Strength and Endurance in Healthy Normals and Elite Male Golfers with and without Low-back Pain," *North American Journal of Sports Physical Therapy*, Vol 1, Iss 2: 80-89, May 2006.

118   Clinical Experience

When I evaluated his downswing, I saw his pelvis drop excessively to the right, his right knee torqued, and he over-pronated his right foot.

In the type of evaluation I perform, I play one area off of the other to see which modification gives me the best result. With this patient, I targeted his pelvis to see if minimizing this compensation resulted in reduced knee pain. Sure enough, when I did this, all of the other areas—including his knee and foot—returned to their normal mechanics and his pain went away. So when he was able to weight shift properly, his knee felt better.

The muscles that were prohibiting him from shifting his weight (during the downswing) were the left external and internal obliques and some of his long back muscles (erector spinae). He did not have any joint stiffness; in fact, he was hypermobile, which means the mobility at his joints was higher than normal.

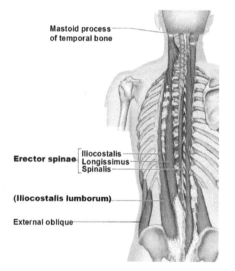

What Worked

To begin, I focused on releasing those muscles that were prohibiting his weight shift. I also evaluated his swing and developed a new strategy so that he could shift his weight from right to left during the downswing.

What I did

- Released the muscles that were prohibiting his weight shift (internal and external obliques, erector spinae)

- Evaluated his golf swing and equalized his weight when he addressed the ball

- Trained a new strategy, incorporating it into the downswing

- Designed exercises to facilitate the proper weight shift and make it more functional, retraining his control

His treatment didn't stop in my office, however. In order to evaluate this golfer in action, I watched his golf lesson, and we worked with his golf coach to get him to equalize his weight when he addressed the ball. They have so many high-tech tools now to analyze your swing and even compare your swing with those of the touring pros, for example. It's great!

I had so much fun watching his golf lesson, so much so that it deepened my belief that merging the worlds of physical therapy and the professional coaching field are absolutely integral to effective assessment and treatment. Having him visually watch his swing and doing a before and after was truly enlightening. He has such a high kinesthetic sense that he was able to correct his pelvis and follow through to the left without knee pain.

"Without question, the art and science of golf takes place in the mind played out through the way we move our bodies. This instinctive connection affects how we feel, how we think and then how we swing our golf club."[119]

Once the muscles were released, and he was able to sense the weight shift to the left without restriction, then we trained a new strategy. He continued to work with the golf pro on this as well. To accomplish this during our treatment sessions, we did a variety of things to incorporate the weight shift and make it functional and fun for him!

Some of these included:

- Ball throws to the left, static throws, and side-stepping throws down a track.

- Side throws against a rebounder (vertical trampoline)

- Balancing on a teeter board

- Side-stepping down a track against resistance, such as a sports cord

- Resisted rotation with a TheraBand

All of these exercises were prescribed in the interest of increasing his awareness of his left side and increasing control during dynamic activities. Once you release the muscles that are holding the old strategy, it is so important to retrain control with the new range of motion gained from the release. I then progressed him through the program and incorporated other corrective exercises when necessary.

It is important to tailor a program that is specific to the **PERSON** and not their body part. That is why knee strengthening, in the case of this golfer, did not make him better. *It only increased his awareness of his right side, which was already heightened.* I believe his history of concussion played into this sense of one-sided dominance. It alters how you move in space as well as your postural awareness.

---

119   Smith, Mark F. Golf Science: Optimum Performance from Tee to Green. University of Chicago Press: 2013.

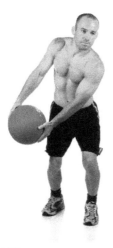

Ball throws left

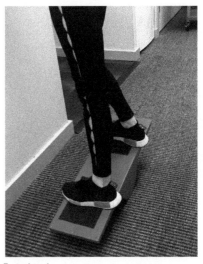

Resisted TheraBand

He could have also done some standing weight shifting on a Pilates reformer or some work on the Cadillac. There are also many yoga poses that could have helped him. However, in the end, I believe a more dynamic program was best suited for him. At the end of the day, it has to be fun for the patient!

It was also vitally important to keep the lines of communication open with his golf coach. After all, we are all on the same team with the same goal!

Teeter board

Positive Results

- Returned to golf pain-free

- Improved his driving distance

- Learned how to control his movement better

- Was able to maximize his workout with his trainer

- Worked more effectively with his golf coach

- Above all, he was having more fun, and that's what it is all about!

Running is a **single leg** activity

Really? My **foot** hurts because I have poor **muscular** control in my **trunk?**

Do foot and heel pain really originate from the foot?

Truth

A chronic or acute foot issue can be a problem within the foot, or the problem could lie somewhere else in the body. Yes, your foot hurts; but is the source of your problem your foot, or is it somewhere else?

If you have had an injury to one side of your body, for example, you tend to put less weight on that side, which could potentially cause problems in the other leg. You end up being treated for a compensation while the source lies elsewhere.

This happens all the time. For example, let's take a closer look at heel pain, a very common issue. Is the problem really your heel, is it plantar fasciitis, or is it something else?[120]

I personally have suffered from heel pain on at least two occasions. Since I live in New York City and walk everywhere, this can be a problem. I also have had patients who have suffered from acute heel pain from some traumatic incident or another and have recovered when their foot was immobilized, which means that they wore a walking boot.[121]

---

120   Lareau, Craig R; Sawyer, Gregory A; Wang, Joanne H; DiGiovanni, Christopher W. "Plantar and Medial Heel Pain: Diagnosis and Treatment." Journal of the American Academy of Orthopaedic Surgeons, Vol 22, Iss 6, 372-380, June 2014.

121   Clinical experience

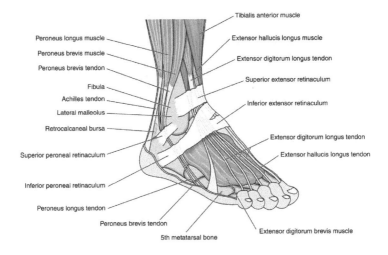

Tibialis anterior muscle
Extensor hallucis longus muscle
Extensor digitorum longus tendon
Superior extensor retinaculum
Inferior extensor retinaculum
Extensor digitorum longus tendon
Extensor hallucis longus tendon
Extensor digitorum brevis muscle
5th metatarsal bone
Peroneus brevis tendon
Peroneus longus tendon
Inferior peroneal retinaculum
Superior peroneal retinaculum
Retrocalcaneal bursa
Lateral malleolus
Achilles tendon
Fibula
Peroneus brevis tendon
Peroneus brevis muscle
Peroneus longus muscle

Pain from a traumatic injury is very different from foot or heel pain that develops without a precipitating incident. You sort of just wake up one day and your heel hurts when you take that first step in the morning. Or perhaps your foot hurts after a long day of walking or a short run in the park. Either way, your foot hurts.

Let's say you hurt your left hip. You immediately offload the hip, which means that you put more weight on your right leg in standing or walking because it feels better. This is a completely natural reaction, but what if you do that for a long time, even after your left hip pain is gone? That would place undue stress on your right side and could possibly leave you with a persistent foot problem that won't go away.[122]

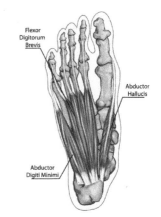

Flexor Digitorum Brevis
Abductor Hallucis
Abductor Digiti Minimi

Consider that you are a runner, like the person in this story. You may have developed a predisposition for running on banked surfaces, or you put more weight on the outside of your foot due to the design of your new running shoes, or you hurt your other foot, hip, or knee years ago and compensated for it by adjusting your running style, and now your other foot hurts.

It sounds like a vicious cycle, doesn't it?

Story

A former patient of mine is a runner who was unfortunately unable to run due to chronic left foot pain. A former marathon runner, he was growing increasingly frustrated with his inability to run without pain. This was going on for about a year. He tried prior physical therapy, orthotics, changing shoes, and injections with little to no relief. His symptoms were localized to his peroneus brevis tendon on the bottom of his foot.

Ironically, walking was not as much of a problem, unless he walked long distances. The mechanical load on the body is far different with running versus walking. I have seen that when people have tried as many interventions as he did without much success, they begin to believe there is no solution or they will never get better.

As a practitioner, I believe that you have simply not found the source of your pain. If it were 100 percent the foot, then he would have gotten better. If you see yourself characterized in this situation, please consider that there may be another source to your problem.

This is what we call "differential diagnosis." There are many sources of heel and foot pain. A *differential diagnosis* is distinguishing a particular disease or condition from others that present similar symptoms.

Think *House*.

In this case a few differential diagnoses include a referral from your spine; it could also be happening from a mechanical overload at the foot, perhaps a peripheral nerve has been affected, it could be because you have some dysfunction in your hips, or it could be that you are not running optimally and placing excessive load on the outside of your foot.[123] The latter is what happened in this story.

---

123   Wille, Christa M; Lenhart, Rachel L; Wang, Sijian; Thelen, Darryl G; Heiderscheit, Bryan C. "Ability of Sagittal Kinematic Variables to Estimate Ground Reaction Forces and Joint Kinetics in Running." Journal of Orthopaedic & Sports Physical Therapy, Vol 44, Iss 10, 625-830: 2014.

What I Found

Since the patient was a runner and running was what provoked his symptoms, I focused on assessing certain components of his running style.

Running is essentially a one-legged activity, therefore looking at his one-legged balance was important. A runner also needs to rotate the torso when running. Most runners display some amount of rotation when they run, from the tight arm hold to a full-blown arm swing.[124]

Sometimes the arm swing is symmetric, where you rotate equally to one side, or it is asymmetric where you over-rotate to one side because of habit or an injury. Either way, they are strategies and in and of themselves not necessarily bad. Again, everyone is different, and my job as the physical therapist is to determine whether the movement is relevant to your injury or movement issue.

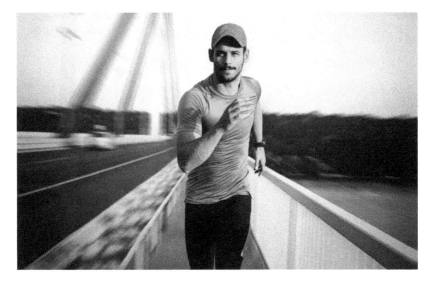

As you can see from this photo, this runner has a nice arm swing, whereas the runners on the next page display minimal rotation with their arms held close to the body, especially the woman on the right.

---

124   Preece, Stephen R; Mason, Duncan; Bramah, Christopher. The Coordinated Movement of the Spine and Pelvis During Running." Human Movement Science, Vol 45, 110-118: Feb 2016.

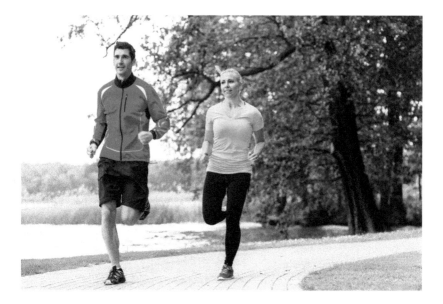

These strategies may work well for different people. There are obvious reasons why people run the way they do. Some feel an arm swing gives them propulsion, while others feel less rotation conserves energy.[125] You can see that the rigidity of your upper body will translate into how you strike your foot and essentially how the body absorbs the shock or the ground reaction force.

We are *heterogeneous*, which means that we are diverse human beings. What works for one person may not work for you. Since we all have different body types, our running and even our walking styles will differ. I am not out to change anyone's running style, I am looking to determine whether or not it is relevant to their story.

My initial evaluation revealed a twist and a lack of control in his foot that was most likely causing the problem. I assessed his single-leg balance as well as a single-leg squat. After all, we do not run with straight knees, so looking at his one-legged mini squat was completely relevant to his problem. I included the arms in the squat, meaning that when he squatted with his left leg, he put his right arm out front. This does simulate the running position to some degree.

---

125   Arellano, Christopher J; Kram, Rodger. The Metabolic Cost of Human Running: Is Swinging the Arms Worth It? Journal of Experimental Biology, Vol 217, 2456-2461: 2014.

As you can see from this image, when this runner is about to place her right foot down, she is rotating her torso to the right and her left arm is out in front.

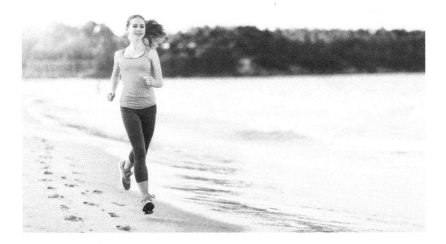

Where was the twist in the patient's foot coming from? Did he just have lousy balance and began using his ankle and foot complex as a strategy to keep upright? Or was that twist being caused by something far from the foot?[126]

What I discovered was when this patient performed a one-legged activity such as a single-leg squat, he shifted his weight to the outside of his left foot, which is exactly where his symptoms presented at his peroneus brevis.

What I also noticed during his evaluation was that as he performed the squat and shifted his weight to the outside of his left foot, he over-rotated his torso to the left, which put more undue pressure on the outside of his foot.

The evaluation also revealed some additional issues going on at his left hip and left knee, but they were not as glaring.

---

126   Park, Jaeyong; Gil Lee, Sang; Bae, Jonglin; Chul Lee, Jung. "The Correlation Between Calcaneal Valgus Angle and Asymmetrical Thoracic- Lumbar Rotation Angles in Patients with Adolescent Scoliosis." Journal of Physical Therapy Science, Vol 27, Iss 12, 3895-3899: Dec 2015.

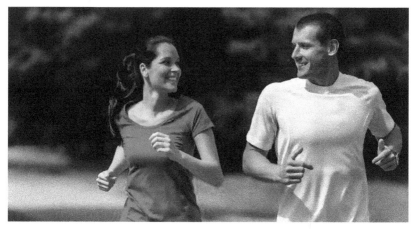

You can see in this photo that each runner has very different rotation patterns as they try to talk to each other.

To further his evaluation, I made some modifications to his one-legged squat until he no longer displayed an excessive shift onto his left foot and his pain was diminished. When I minimized his over-rotation to the left in his torso, his foot mechanics were better, and he felt better as well. It is no surprise that when I tested his trunk rotation to the right, he was limited.

Additionally, when I watched him run, I noted the same increased rotation and backward arm movement on his left side. What does this mean? When he ran, his left elbow extended further back than his right elbow, which caused an over-rotation on his left side. The result? It put increased pressure on the outside of his left foot while running. Our nervous system adjusts our movement over time, and ultimately this was his current strategy.

To be clear, some people run fine this way. And there are others—whose bodies have reached their buckle point or threshold—who don't.

There were certain muscles that were causing his over-rotation as well as some imbalances in his foot that needed to be addressed. Since this was such a persistent problem, the foot needed to be treated at some point, albeit secondarily.

If you have read other parts of this book, you will notice similar muscle groups as culprits when it comes to over- or under-rotating the torso. For example, external and internal obliques are big trunk rotators.

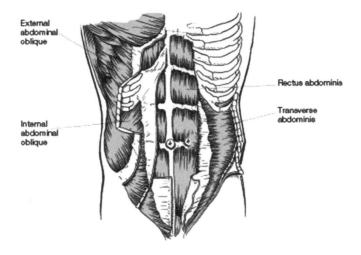

External abdominal oblique

Internal abdominal oblique

Rectus abdominis

Transverse abdominis

What Worked

As a result of my evaluation, I found that he needed to have the over-rotation in his thorax and subsequent foot imbalances corrected.

What I did

- Released certain trunk muscles (external & internal obliques) that contributed to this over-rotation (Remember in the other foot story that this was a similar problem?)

- Trained a new strategy once these muscles were freed up

- Increase his right trunk (thoracic) rotation

- Corrective physical therapy exercises to normalize his movement and rotation so that he could run without foot pain

- Change body schema to increase awareness of right side in brain

- Treated the foot imbalances (detailed treatment below)

To begin treatment, I released the muscles in his mid-back and abdomen that were contributing to this excessive left thoracic rotation. Through my assessment, I found that he needed to control his trunk once these muscles were freed up. Though his treatment did include muscle release, he was not stiff, so he did not require joint mobilization or stretching. Stretching may feel good, but if it is not what you need, you are only giving in to the problem.

What he needed was to open up the right side of his trunk in order to equalize his left and right rotation. Once again, I'll repeat, you DON'T need to have equal rotation to both sides to run well. However, in this story, it was one of the main reasons his foot pain persisted. Remember, we are training your brain by giving it different options for movement.

We had to change his body schema as well as increase awareness of his right side in his brain. Remember that your body parts have a representation in certain parts of your brain.[127]

---

127   Bracci, Stefania; Caramazza, Alfonso; Peelen, Marius. "Representational Similarity of Body Parts in Human Occipitotemporal Cortex." Journal of Neuroscience, Vol 35, Iss 38, 12977-12985: Sept 2015.

The plan to increase awareness of his right side included right lateral lunges, one-legged stance activities with rotation right, as well as one-legged squats and lunges with rotation. Remember that running is a one-legged activity. If you don't train on one leg, you are missing an important piece in your rehab as well as your training program.

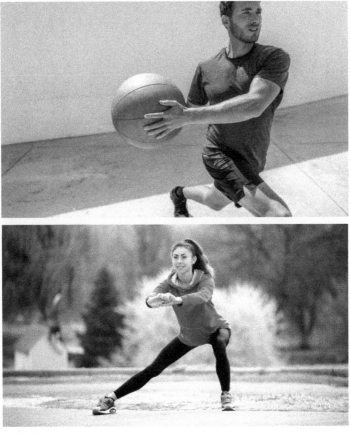

Lateral lunge

The lateral lunge increases your body awareness of one side over the other and also helps train both sides of your body and brain. We then incorporated rotation with the lunge, as it was a huge issue for this patient. I think by now you must agree that rotation is an important component for running as well as life, right? We function in multiple planes, and rotation is one of those motions that we need in 3D!

We could also have done some yoga poses, such as the half-moon pose with rotation. This pose opens up the rib cage on the side that is facing up.

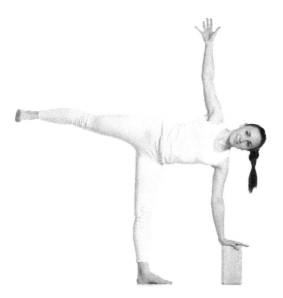

This would train the one-legged component as well as rotation. Your imagination is the only barrier here. In addition to releasing the muscles that caused the over-rotation and retraining body awareness of the right side through one-legged movements with rotation, we addressed the initial patient complaint—the foot. We treated the foot, as it was a contributing source to the problem. However, treating the foot alone would not have made it fully better, as he had experienced in the past with unsuccessful treatments. He needed someone to address the missing piece to the puzzle—the actual *cause* of the foot pain.

What I did

- Manual therapy to the foot and ankle area

- Nerve glides to increase the mobility of some of the nerves in the foot that tend to get exacerbated when the foot becomes chronic

- Stabilization training to increase control and even out the distribution of forces across the foot

- Specific releases to the muscles of his foot that were gripping and holding his foot in positions that were non-optimal

- There are many other treatment options, but these were the ones that I chose at that time based on his presentation.

In working with the patient to optimize his rotation while running, we were able to make the foot treatment finally "stick."

Positive Results

- His running and running time improved!

- He was able to achieve his goal of running another marathon!

- He also learned that there are other body parts to consider while searching for a solution to his foot pain while running.

- Most importantly, he now has the knowledge to prevent this from happening again.

Mindful movement helps create new brain maps

Really? My **foot** continues to hurt because of an overactive **abdominal muscle**?

Did you know that the answer to your foot pain may not lie in your foot?

Truth

At this point in the book, I think you may realize that I am all about thinking outside of the box. Don't get me wrong—foot pain can come from the foot. But when you have a symptom that is not going away despite continued treatment to the area, you really have to look at other options. Sure, that foot may need to get treated, but it is SECONDARY in these cases. It is all about getting the right treatment at the right time.

Our feet are the basis for our weight shifting, our balance, our walking, and basically anything we do upright or vertical. There is a functional interplay between the foot and other parts of our body.

It has been shown in the research that decreased postural stability has been linked to abnormal foot mechanics.[128] This is not surprising. Depending on the potential loss of balance, the body employs an ankle strategy to keep us from falling. If the perturbation is forceful enough, then the body starts to stabilize itself via other mechanisms.

---

128   Cobb, Stephen C; Bazett-Jones, David M; Joshi, Mukta M; Earl Boehm, Jennifer E; James, Roger C. "The Relationship Among Foot Posture, Core and Lower Extremity Muscle Function, and Postural Stability." Journal of Athletic Training, Vol 49, Iss 2, 173-180: Mar-Apr 2014.

And if that ankle has sustained an injury, whether it be chronic or acute, our body naturally offloads that injury by increasing the weight on the other foot. We have all been there: we sprain our ankles, start limping, thereby putting less weight on the injured side, naturally. Our nervous system makes a decision regarding where we put our weight. The injured foot or the other foot? How we place our foot or how much weight we put on it will influence postural control.[129]

Our center of mass shifts, and then we develop compensations over time that help us function better initially. However, after the injury heals, it is these persistent compensatory mechanisms that end up feeding back into the initial injury. These are old strategies that need to be replaced by new ones—similar to developing a new habit.

For example, if you have an injury to your right foot, you will put more weight on your left foot to feel better. It's that simple. Over time, when your injury has healed, you may still put more weight on the other foot due to that learned response. Those compensatory mechanisms must be unlearned and retrained, or they may affect how you move, especially if you are performing repetitive movement over and over again. This was the case in this person's story.

Story

One of my patients had a chronic right foot problem, which resulted in her having a PRP (Platelet-Rich Plasma) injection into her symptomatic posterior tibialis tendon.

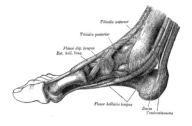

PRP is produced from a person's own blood. It is a concentration of one type of cell, known as platelets, which circulate through the blood and are critical for blood clotting. Platelets and the liquid plasma portion of the blood contain many factors that are essential for the cell recruitment, multiplication,

---

129   Zhou, J; Ning, X, Hu, B; Dai, B. "The influences of foot placement on lumbopelvic rhythm during trunk flexion motion." Journal of Biomechanics, Apr 2016.

and specialization that are required for healing.[130]

There is some positive evidence currently as to the efficacy of these injections, however more research is needed to determine their long-term value and their overall effectiveness in humans.[131,132] In this instance, the PRP injections healed her tendon but did not heal her.

Still unable to walk long distances, go up into a ballet relevé position (below), or even weight shift and balance onto her right leg without pain, she was getting frustrated. She had physical therapy somewhere else with no significant relief.

When I saw her for the first time, she was concerned at her lack of progress and was growing increasingly discouraged that she would never be able to function in the way that she was used to. Her occupation as an actor in a Broadway show required her to sustain multiple hours on her feet with a multitude of costume changes. And to top it all off, she had to wear a corset underneath all those layers of clothing!

When I evaluated her relevé, the symptoms in her right foot were set off the minute she moved forward onto her toes. The same thing happened with the weight shift onto her right leg, not to mention balancing on her right leg as well.

It was clear that we would need to address all of these components as part of her overall treatment plan, especially considering the great physical demands of her job.

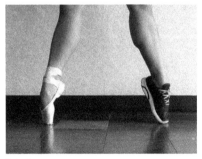

Relevé

Many would think that going up on your toes is a task that is seemingly straightforward and

---

130 For more information please see http://orthoinfo.aaos.org/topic.cfm?topic=A00648.

131 Moraes, VY; Lenza, M; Tamaoki, MJ; Faloppa, F; Belloti, JC. "Platelet-rich therapies for musculoskeletal soft tissue injuries." Cochrane Database Syst Rev 2013 Dec 23; (12).

132 Gormeli, Gokay, et. al. "Multiple PRP injections are more effective than single injections and hyaluronic acid in knees with early osteoarthritis: a randomized, double-blind, placebo-controlled trial." KSSTA, March 2017, Vol 25, Iss 3, pp 958-965.

symmetrical. Try doing that without holding onto something—and while carrying, minimally, twenty five pounds of costume in your left hand. It would not feel so easy and symmetrical then, would it? As a matter of fact, that is one of the movements this person had to perform in her show. Not to mention the constant pivoting on her feet while carrying as well.

The more load and repetition you add to an activity, the more precise and synchronous your movements have to be. Performing calf raises in a gym once a week is relatively mild compared to the repetitive nature of an activity done multiple times over a course of several performances.

In addition, with her not having been able to work for quite some time now, one can only imagine the emotional issues also playing into the presentation. These MUST be addressed for the person to achieve lasting change and not just some short-term relief that does her no service at all.

Pain education and compassion go a long way here.[133,134,135]

What I Found

Since weight shifting onto her right leg was a problem and the "easier" of her tasks (versus the relevé), we started there. Given all the physical requirements of her performance, I believed a gross assessment of her baseline posture in standing to be important to developing an effective treatment plan for her. I think of baseline posture checks as a standard check that airline pilots or racecar drivers do before they start their engines. Kind of important, don't you think?

She undoubtedly had some issues in her feet, a flattened arch, a dropped rear foot, which were worse on her right.

But the most noticeable piece was the increased weight bearing on her left foot and a rotation in her trunk to the right. At that point, this was most likely a

---

133   Bunzil, Samantha; McEvoy, Sarah; DanKaerts, Wim; O'Sullivan, Peter; O'Sullivan, Kieran. "Patient Perspectives on Participation in Cognitive Functional Therapy for Chronic Low-back Pain." Cognitive Behavior Therapy & Pain, Sept 2016.

134   Fersum, K. Vibe; O'Sullivan, P; Skouen, JS; Smith, A; Kvale, A. "Efficacy of classification-based cognitive functional therapy in patients with non-specific chronic low-back pain: A randomized controlled trial." European Journal of Pain, Vol 17, Iss 6, 916-928: July 2013.

135   Mosely, G. Lorimer; Butler, David S. "Fifteen Years of Explaining Pain: The Past, Present, and Future." The Journal of Pain, Vol 16, Iss 9, 807-813: Sept 2015.

learned response, as I mentioned previously. So in order for her to equalize her weight bearing and balance appropriately, she had to work really hard.

EXERCISE: You try it. Stand with more weight on your left foot and then rotate to the right, noticing what happens to your right foot. Imagine doing this day after day. The stress and strain it puts on the posterior tibialis may increase if you cannot adjust your position.[136]

Along with the increased weight shift came all the other compensations: the left hip, right foot (of course) and knee, then the head, neck, and trunk just so her gaze could be straightforward.

The body takes the path of least resistance. It says, "How can I achieve my goal with the least amount of opposition?" This happens especially in the milliseconds it requires to shift your weight from one foot to the other.

When she shifted her weight to the right, the rotation in her thorax became much worse, as did all the other compensations mentioned above, and, as a result, her symptoms increased. When I played one area off of the other, the modification that made her feel the best was the change I made to her thorax. By change, I mean giving her body the option, manually, to get more of her weight on to her right foot without pain. Once again, I gave her nervous system a better option. When I say *best*, I mean pain-free with an optimal movement pattern. That, of course, varies with everyone and is one of the reasons why your initial evaluation should be tailored to you and the specific movements associated with your symptoms.

I then assessed her relevé. I saw the same pattern—left trunk shift and rotation to the right. When someone has a persistent problem, you tend to see the same dominant movement pattern and strategy across all activities. It is not surprising that she had limited trunk rotation to the left when I tested it. (Remember, most of the rotation in the back comes from your thorax.)

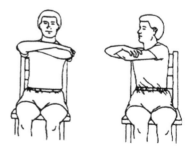

---

136 Clinical Experience

Having said this, since her foot pain was so persistent for such a long time, it most likely was a secondary cause of her problem and needed to be addressed. However, treating the foot by itself would offer no lasting relief, as she experienced previously with the short-term and limited relief of the PRP injections and prior PT.

In order to address the source of her issues, I needed to get to the bottom of why she continued to place most of her weight on her left foot. What was causing it? Looking at the demands of her performance, it was clear that the asymmetrical nature of her requirements on stage caused her to overuse certain muscles in her trunk, creating imbalances in control and force production. And this, in turn, trickled down to her foot, which was already sore and overworked.

Imagine holding a twenty-five-pound weight in your left hand while performing your general daily activities like squatting, bending, etc. How do you, in effect, stabilize yourself? What muscles would you use? You could use external and/or internal obliques (page 193). And they attach to the thorax. It is no surprise that when chronically overworked, as in this story, they caused imbalances in her trunk, which then trickled down to her foot.

What Worked

Due to the persistent and long-term nature of her foot pain, I needed to address what I felt to be the primary source of her problem—the thorax—first and the foot second.

What I did

- Introduction of Recognise™[137]App for rehab and to reduce flare-ups

- Address the sensitized issues in her foot via Mirror Box Therapy[138]

- Mirror Box Therapy was initially used to relieve symptoms associated with phantom limb pain. It has since been shown to be effective in reducing symptoms in persistent pain syndromes.[139]

- Muscle releases were performed to the left external oblique and diaphragm. Remember those stabilization strategies? Sometimes we overwork certain muscles and then we do not know how to turn them off.

- Oscillatory joint mobilizations to her mid thorax to dampen down muscle activation

- Taping to help support her thorax and increase her ability to control her movement, particularly rotation (see page 194 for photo)

- Taping of foot initially to reinforce the new desired movement pattern (see page 113 for photo)

- Child's pose to open up the rib cage

- Weight shifting onto her right foot, progressing to full weight bearing to one-legged balance

- Side-lying trunk openers (also known as book covers) and focused step forward walks

---

137   http://www.noigroup.com/en/product/btrapp

138   Ramachandran, V. S., Rogers-Ramachandran, D. C. Synaesthesia in phantom limbs induced with mirrors, Proceedings of the Royal Society of London 1996; (263(1369)):37 7-386,doi: 10.1098/rspb.1996.00SS, PMID 8637922.

139 Frederik J. A. Deconinck, PhD, et al. "Reflections on Mirror Therapy: A Systematic Review of the Effect of Mirror Visual Feedback on the Brain." Neurorehabilitation and Neural Repair. 2015, Vol 29, Issue 4, pp. 349-361.

I felt it was important to address the sensitized tissues in her foot first via the use of a Mirror Box. It is extremely helpful for desensitizing a heightened nervous system that has experienced long-term, persistent pain. It is also a really nice, non-threatening way to validate a person's symptoms and allow progression of treatment. Think of it as training your brain with a mirror.

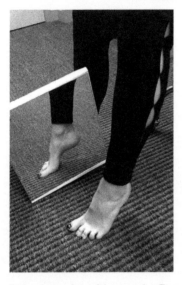

Mirror Box Training is also part of an integrated approach to pain called Greater Motor Imagery (GMI).[140,141] GMI was developed initially for an application to chronic limb pain. For more on this approach, please see http://www.gradedmotorimagery.com. It certainly is engaging and fun! I have found that the Mirror Box is also useful for calming down acute flare-ups. For this patient, we started with gentle movements of her uninvolved (left) side progressing to sitting calf raises.

I also introduced her to the Recognise App developed by NOI Group of Australia.[142] She used the app as part of her rehab process and also when she had an acute flare-up. The ability to recognize a part of the body as belonging or moving to the left or the right involves brain processes that are important for normal function. In some situations, for example after injury, the ability to recognize body parts and movements as being left or

140   http://www.gradedmotorimagery.com/; http://www.noigroup.com/en/Product/BTGMIB

141   The Graded Motor Imagery Handbook Lorimer Moseley, David Butler, Timothy Beames, Thomas Giles NOI Group, 2012.

142   http://www.noigroup.com/recognise

right becomes reduced.[143,144] For more information, visit the NOI Group website at http://www.noigroup.com/recognise. This was very helpful for when she flared up.

Soft tissue releases were performed to the left external oblique and diaphragm as well as oscillatory joint mobilizations to her mid-thorax to dampen down muscle activation. These are manual, hands-on techniques used to increase mobility of a given muscle or joint or to reduce overactive tone in a particular part of the body. As you can see from the photo below, the external oblique is an important abdominal muscle, which when activated increases trunk rotation to the opposite side. The left external oblique reinforces right trunk rotation.

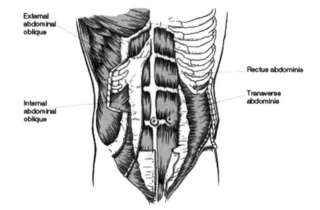

The diaphragm is an important respiratory muscle, and when it is put in a compromised position, it can affect your ability to breathe, to open up your rib cage, and your voice carry (which is important for an actor), as well as a host of other issues not relevant to this person's story. In her case, I believe the limited ability of her diaphragm to expand was caused by the

143   Linder M, Michaelson P, Röijezon U. Laterality judgments in people with low-back pain- A cross-sectional observational and test-retest reliability study. *Man Ther* 2016;21: 128-133.

144 Breckenridge, JD et al. "The development of a shoulder specific left/right judgement task: Validity & reliability." *Musculoskeletal Science & Practice*. 2017 Apr; 28:39-45. doi: 10.1016/j. msksp.2017.01.009. Epub 2017 Jan 27.

overworked external oblique muscle, which affected her ability to rotate her trunk. I believe this was due to the constant pivoting and bending that she had to do in the show. And to top it all off, she was carrying items that weighed about twenty-five pounds. Talk about control!

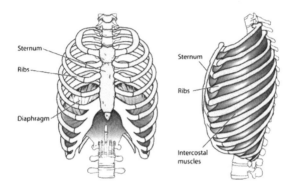

Thoracic cage

I used tape to help support her thorax (see below) and increase her ability to control her movement, particularly rotation.[145] She has told me that this helped her quite a bit, not just for the support but for the tactile feedback she got when she happened to fall back to her old strategy. (Note: I did also tape her foot at one point to reinforce the new movement pattern we wanted.)

Remember, she wears a corset in the show, and they are quite compressive. *When clinical reasoning shows that decompression is what is needed here, it is no wonder that wearing the corset made her worse!*

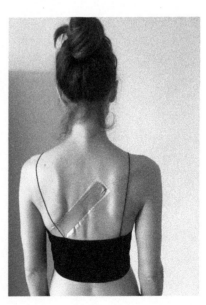

---

145   Lee, Diane and Lee, Linda Joy (LJ). *Discover Physio Series*, Vancouver, B.C., 2012.

At the end of the day, it is all about how you move. Physiotherapists are experts at movement analysis, and helping you move better is what we do best. Making movement less threatening to your nervous system is one of the ultimate goals. In order for her to open her rib cage, I gave her the child's pose. If you are reading the whole book, you will notice that this is one of my "go-to" postures to decompress the trunk.

We also did some weight shifting onto her right foot, progressing to full weight bearing to one-legged balance. These were done with specific cues. A couple of hers were the following: "Imagine you have balloons in your arm pits"[146] or "Imagine you have a pile of dominoes, and all the dominoes are stacked one on top of the other."

These cues are specific to her, but certainly helped as she is a visual learner and was able to sync the images in her brain with the movement. Many of my patients use these types of cues and find them very helpful. Remember, you are training your brain as well as your body.

She also did side-lying "book covers" to the left (these are mentioned in a previous case on page 148), as well as focused step forward walks with rotation left. This is a movement pattern we needed to reinforce.

A progression of this included the addition of weights, as she needed to do this for her show. We started her lying on her back with her knees bent doing basic resistance exercises such as triceps extensions and reverse flyes. These were all done with the cues that were mentioned above.

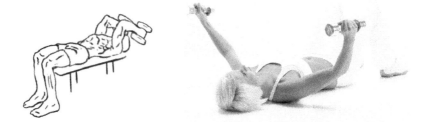

---

146   Lee, Diane and Lee, Linda Joy (LJ). *Discover Physio Series*, Vancouver, B.C., 2012.

As you can see, it is all about relating treatment specifically to a movement she was having problems with (relevé). Again, I cannot emphasize enough the importance of tailoring a program that is specific to your needs. Once that was remastered, we worked on combined movements she had to do on stage. For example, standing and pivoting on her leg, going up stairs with weight in her arms, as well as hopping on stage.

We could have incorporated Pilates or yoga into the program as well. This patient was extremely compliant with her home program, and it is to her credit that she progressed along as she did.

Positive Results

The good news is that she is back to work! We have substituted a Spanx® Tank for the corset. (Remember we want decompression here, not compression and Spanx is less compressing than wearing a corset!!) She is able to wear her show shoes, and can walk longer distances outside. In addition, her relevé and balance are normal now. She can also manage the loads her job requires—particularly carrying the weight, costumes, etc. on stage—without a problem.

And I think most important is that she has a sense of hope and assurance that she can confidently move forward without the fear that she will ever be debilitated by this issue again. Knowledge is power, education is strength, and courage is looking head-on and knowing that you can manage anything you set your mind to. Even foot pain.

Healing starts with someone **listening to your story**

Chapter 15

Really? My **wrist** pain is coming from my **shoulder**?

Did you know that wrist pain could originate in your shoulder complex? Sounds strange? Wrist pain is wrist pain, right? Not always.

Truth

Short of a fall on an outstretched arm or wrist pain induced from a repetitive strain injury (and even that may originate somewhere else), wrist pain can have an insidious, unknown onset.

You have seen people with wrist splints on—they are trying to immobilize the joint in order for it to heal. Splints are very helpful when it comes to wrist pain.[147] But after the splint is taken off and the person goes back to normal activity, the wrist pain may return. If that is the case, then it begs the question: What caused it?

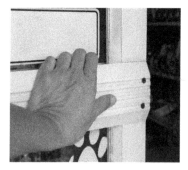

We never think of the wrist, or the hand for that matter, as a weight-bearing joint. But it is. Many people use their hands and wrists to stand up.

Or to do a push-up, open a door, or do a down dog in yoga.

One could always modify certain painful activities in the interim, espe-

---

147   http://www.ncbi.nlm.nih.gov/pubmedhealth/PMH0072780/

cially if it is the non-dominant hand. That is hard to do for some people, but the brain (and nervous system) figures a way to do it.

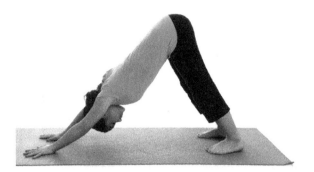

In the above photo of downward-facing dog, you can see that the more you throw your body weight forward, the more pressure it puts on your wrists. If someone has sustained an injury to their wrist, this position could potentially aggravate it if not properly rehabbed.

Furthermore, since this position is a full-body movement and requires the interplay of multiple joints and muscles, any compensation resulting from an injury could result in poor form, thus perpetuating the issue.

Story

A patient of mine sustained an injury to her right wrist while lifting a heavy box. She felt something "go" in her wrist, and it was sore from then on. At the advice of her physician, she put a splint on it and rested. Pertinent recreational history included Pilates and yoga. She was also right-hand dominant.

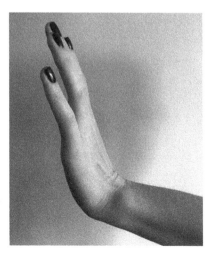

As a result of her injury, she could not actively extend her wrist (see photo), lift heavy objects, or do any gripping.

Since she did yoga, this was a problem for her, as she could not move forward onto her hands to get into a full down dog. Another limitation existed in her job, as it also required her to do some lifting.

Down dog is a fairly symmetrical posture, and if one imposes an asymmetrical force or position upon it, then the body will adapt in some way—by taking away or adding motion to another body part.

For example, you can see that if one shoulder is forward in this posture, it will likely place extra pressure on the wrist. You try it: go into down dog and turn your shoulder girdle to the left.

Imagine your upper body is turned to the left for some reason (could be from tight right pectoral (chest) muscles or something else pulling to the left); the right wrist has to adapt to that force naturally in this weight-bearing posture.

Downward-facing dog is what we call a closed chain exercise—those performed where the hands or feet are fixed in space and cannot move. The extremity remains in constant contact with the immobile surface, usually the ground or the base of a machine. So, by default, if you change the position of one joint in a closed-chain exercise like downward-facing dog, there will be effects up and down the chain, so to speak.

So in this position, for example, if you shift your hips to the left, you can feel the effects of this shift on other body parts. This is a simple example, but imagine effecting this type of movement over and over again, then your body becomes used to it. And now you have a new movement pattern—a new "normal," so to speak.

What I Found

When I saw this patient for the initial consultation, she was still wearing the splint occasionally while working. She could not weight bear on her wrist or perform full, active wrist extension without pain. Since she did yoga, she told me she could not do the down dog or any other weight-bearing posture, for that matter.

Her baseline position showed a forward and anterior right shoulder, and her shoulder girdle was rotated to the left. This is not surprising, since she is right-handed.

When I had her perform the down dog, I did notice that she was putting more weight on her right arm, which was unusual because the brain usually offloads the painful side. This obviously provoked her symptoms. Not only was she putting more weight on her right arm, but her right shoulder moved further forward into the posture.

Bear in mind that the shoulder, elbow, wrist, and hand all work together. The interdependence of these structures and the nerve innervation that they share is important when distinguishing the causes of upper extremity pain.

Why was she putting more weight onto the right arm? It was likely that she had always put more weight on her right arm and hand, but since her wrist was aggravated due to injury, that extra weight shift now gave her pain.

When I had her try and adjust her posture to bring the shoulder back, she felt better and her wrist was able to extend more into the pose. When I manually brought her shoulder back, I felt this strong resistance coming from the front of her chest and into the upper ribs. This was most likely a muscle imbalance.

Interestingly, when she lay on her back on the table, and I manually re-positioned the shoulder, her wrist extension improved then!

I had found the insidious cause of her wrist pain!

What Worked

After that discovery during the evaluation, I naturally directed the majority of treatment to her shoulder. Don't get me wrong—I did also treat her wrist, as this was still somewhat of an acute issue.

What I did

- Soft tissue release to pectoralis minor and second and third intercostal muscles (Intercostal muscles are situated between the ribs.)

- Manual therapy to shoulder complex

- Breath work to help desensitize tissues

- Pectoral muscle stretches (performed at home)

- Yoga and Pilates postures to open up the chest and upper rib cage

- Lifting techniques to support the wrist

I believe that the muscles holding her shoulder in that pattern were the pectoral muscles (particularly, pec minor) and the second and third intercostal muscles (not shown).

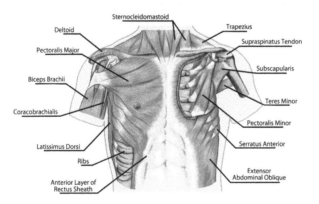

Simply put, one of the functions of the pec minor is that it raises the upper ribs during inspiration (breathing in) and stabilizes the shoulder blade (scapula). When it is overactive, it can draw the shoulder complex forward and elevate the ribs.

Soft tissue release was done to those muscles as well as manual therapy to her shoulder complex. This is all done in an effort to dampen down the tone in these muscles. Remember that increased tone in a muscle is a result of increased neural drive to those muscles from the brain.

We also did some breath work, which also helped desensitize the tissues.[148, 149] Stretches for the pectoral muscles were done at home. See the most common pectoral stretches below:

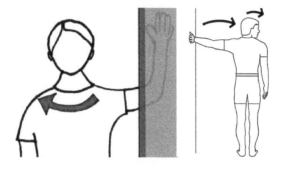

Although she did not have a nerve injury, we also did some neural mobilizations to increase the mobility of the structures in her upper arm. It is all about getting the blood flowing so the arm can move better, and it's fun!

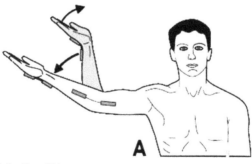

Median Nerve Glide

---

148   Doran, Natasha J. "Experiencing Wellness within Illness: Exploring a Mindfulness-Based Approach to Chronic Back Pain." Qualitative Health Research, Vol 24, Iss 6, 749-760: June 2014.

149   Victoria, Himmat Kaur; Caldwell, Christine. "Breathwork in Body Psychotherapy : Clinical Applications." Body, Movement and Dance in Psychotherapy, Vol 8, Iss 4: 2013.

Additionally, some yoga postures to open up the chest and upper rib cage are triangle pose and lateral angle pose. She was doing Pilates, so she incorporated upper chest openers into her program.

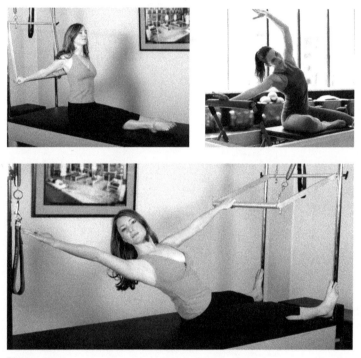

Pilates exercises

These are just a few samples of what you can do.

You can also progress to modified weight-bearing postures, such as down dog against the wall (see image next page) and then eventually a full down dog.

We also worked on some lifting techniques to support her wrist so she could try and prevent this injury from reoccurring.

At the end of the day, it is all about movement, and particularly the movement that is relevant for you. As I've said time and again, what works for you may not work for someone else, and vice versa.

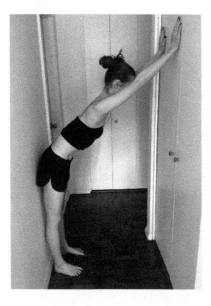

Positive Results

Her wrist pain went away, and she was able to lift, do yoga, and Pilates. In the end, that's what it's all about—regaining the ability to do the activities and movements you love to do!

A society
that treats
symptoms,
not **causes**, is a
society that
is **clueless**

Chapter 16

Really? My **elbow** STILL hurts because of an issue with my **neck** and **shoulder**?

Isn't it frustrating when you have chronic elbow pain? You feel like it will never go away. Especially if it comes back after your elbow has been treated. And, even worse, you do not play tennis or golf!

Truth

Elbow pain is extremely common. As a matter of fact, up to 3 percent of the general population will experience elbow pain at some point in their lives. Even more so (64 percent) when you perform an occupation with repetitive manual tasks, or play a sport that requires repetitive gripping like tennis or golf. Hence, the terms golfer's or tennis elbow.[150]

But there are many people who have elbow pain who do not play those sports at all. Several years ago, I experienced elbow pain. I chalked it up to all the hands-on work that I do. At that time, I was playing more golf, so that was a factor I am sure.

The elbow is primarily a hinge joint (it bends and straightens), but it also possesses the ability to rotate the forearm into pronation and supination. Golf and tennis are obviously rotary sports, which is why this condition tends to get associated with them.

---

150   Shiri, R; Viikari-Juntura, E.; Varonen, H.; Heliövarre, M., Prevalence and determinants of lateral and medial epicondylitis: a Population Study," American Journal of Epidemiology, Vol 164, Iss 11: 1065-74, Dec 2006.

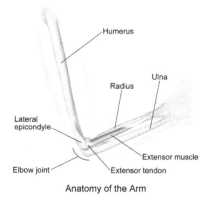

Anatomy of the Arm

However, if you have a shoulder that is limited in rotation, whether it's internal or external rotation, you will tend to compensate further down the chain, which in this case is the elbow.[151] For example, if you have limited internal rotation of your shoulder, you will compensate with your forearm in golf when you are following through with the club. This motion of internal rotation and its associated muscles help you power through the ball on your way to a great shot!

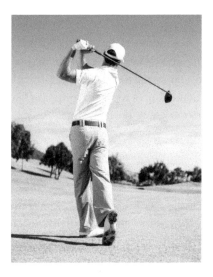

But if you have a limitation in your shoulder, the body looks somewhere else to get that movement. The next joint down is the elbow complex. So what does the body do? Or simply put, how does your nervous system adjust to hit that great shot? It may increase the rotational torque in your forearm to the muscles that power the club through. Do that over and over again, and you could potentially be setting yourself up for an elbow problem.

How would you know that you had this limited motion in your

151   Shitara, H., Kobayashi, T., Yamamoto, A. et al. "Prospective multifactorial analysis of preseason risk factors for shoulder and elbow injuries in high school baseball pitchers," Knee Surg Sports Traumatol Arthrosc (2015). doi:10.1007/s00167-015-3731-4.

shoulder? You would not, really. That is why I think it is so important to see a physical therapist before starting any new sport or exercise program. Prevention is what you want here.

Additionally, if you have limitations in your wrist or forearm, you will compensate further up the arm, which is the elbow. Or if you have had an injury to one of the ligaments in your elbow, you will try and stabilize the elbow with another compensatory muscle or ligament. Ultimately, what we need to do is change your strategy.

Or in the case with my patient, he had a history of neck pain, which caused him to compensate at his shoulder, which then caused him to compensate at the lateral elbow. A double whammy! Everybody has a different buckle point, that's what makes us so unique![152]

Story

A patient of mine was a news producer here in NYC. He had a high stress job—a lot of sitting, a lot of computer time, as well as a lot of reading. He did not play golf or tennis, ironically. But he did work out twice a week with a trainer. Thankfully! Stress needs some release.

One day, he was doing some heavy biceps curls and noticed that after the workout, his elbow was sore when he had to grip or carry something. Had he reached his buckle point? Did something give in his system? Maybe, maybe not. But his elbow hurt and that was that.

He did not think anything of it and figured it would go away. It was also his dominant arm. Note: In my clinical experience, elbow pain rarely goes away on its own. And if it does, it takes a while. Most people wait to see if it does, then when it doesn't, they seek help for it. If I can impart one word of advice here: DON'T WAIT. This is one thing that generally gets worse if you don't get it looked at.

He really enjoyed working out and did not want to take a break, so we had to modify some of the workouts. Every time he went to pick up a dumbbell, his elbow hurt.

---

152   Lee, A. T., & Lee-Robinson, A. L. (2010). The Prevalence of Medial Epicondylitis Among Patients With C6 and C7 Radiculopathy. *Sports Health*, 2(4), 334–336. http://doi.org/10.1177/1941738109357304.

As I mentioned in the introduction of this book, I have sustained many an injury over the years, but I have always tried to do some activity. As of this writing, I have a hip problem I am dealing with. Too many stairs in Rome last summer! However, I am continuing to go to spin class because it does not bother me when I spin. The benefits far outweigh the risks here.

Think about it: when you have to carry something heavy in your hand, push or pull a heavy object, or pick up something heavy repeatedly, that movement produces a lot of force through your elbow joint. Try and keep the object close to your body, that way it shortens the lever arm and minimizes the forces going through your elbow joint.

> "I believe that my patients should still work out with their personal trainers. It just takes some modifications and a little creativity! No excuses here, my friends."

This type of movement requires not just a lot of biceps, but a lot of shoulder and scapular action as well. If you only used your elbow muscles to repeatedly pick up something, and not your rhomboids, deltoid, etc., then you would be setting yourself up for a potential muscle imbalance.

I once treated a semi-professional tennis player with the largest fore-arms I have ever seen. Her shoulder muscles were so weak—no wonder she had to use another strategy. Not surprisingly, she came to me with elbow pain.

Remember: You do the same thing over and over again, you get the same thing you've always gotten: pain and dysfunction. This is true even for professional athletes who are the best compensators of them all.

What I Found

If you have read some of the other stories in the book, you know the type of evaluation I perform. A full body assessment. I know you are prob-ably thinking, *Elbow? Are you kidding me?* Trust me, if you have had elbow pain for a long time, you'll want your physical therapist to look to the moon if they could. Because you want this elbow pain gone yesterday, right? I know I did.

For starters, his elbow was sore, and repeated elbow and wrist movements did reproduce his symptoms, for sure. But this was secondary. And of course, we did treat it. But not as much as another area.

When I evaluated his neck (cervical spine) movements, I noticed a significant restriction in his upper neck. This is quite common in people who sit a lot and tend to lean forward to look at their computers and down to look at their smartphones. It is what it is. Until a threshold is reached, then compensations start to happen.

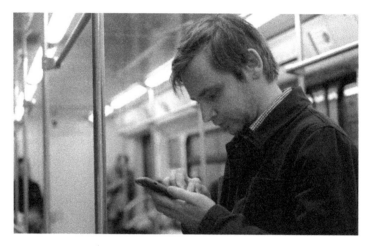

As I progressed through the evaluation of his neck, I noticed that when I assessed his lower cervical spine, C5-7, the 5th through 7th cervical vertebrae, I reproduced his elbow symptoms.[153] See the photo on the following page for a description and picture of the relevant anatomy.

What?

The nerve supply to the elbow comes from the neck. That is the human body.

---

153   Berglund KM, Persson BH, Denison E. "Prevalence of pain and dysfunction in the cervical and thoracic spine in persons with and without lateral elbow pain," *Manual Therapy*, Vol 13, Iss 4, Aug 2008.

Dermatome Map of the
Upper Limb (Anterior View)

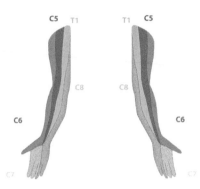

A dermatome is an area of the skin supplied by
nerves from a single spinal root.

For some reason, when I palpated his lower neck, his symptoms were reproduced. Important finding to be sure. My guess, or hypothesis, was that under normal circumstances the neck would be inconsequential, BUT given the buildup of excess computer work, stress, lack of sleep, and possibly some immune issues (he was sick for a while with a prolonged cold), this resulted in his body reacting the way it did. Go figure.[154,155]

A common clinical pattern that I see is a restriction in the upper cervical spine (C1 and C2, also known as the atlas and axis) with excess mobility further down (C5,6). And sometimes structures (bone, muscle, etc.) that are innervated[156] by C5-6 can possibly get cranky, which is my non-technical term for irritated. Note from the image above that the elbow is innervated from C6. That's why persistent elbow pain, and persistent pain in general, deserve a different approach. Wouldn't you agree?

---

154   Koffel, Erin; Kroenke, Kurt; Bair, Matthew J.; Leverty, David; Polusny, Melissa A.; Krebs, Erin E., "The bidirectional relationship between sleep complaints and pain: Analysis of data from a randomized trial." Health Psychology, Vol 35(1), Jan 2016, 41-49. http://dx.doi. org/10.1037/hea0000245

155   Marchand, F.; Perretti, M.; McMahon, S.B.; "The role of the immune system in chronic pain," Health Psychology Vol 35, Iss 1: 41-49. Jan 2016.

156   Innervated means *receives nerve supply from*. These structures receive their nerve supply from the 5th and 6th cervical vertebrae (C5-C6).

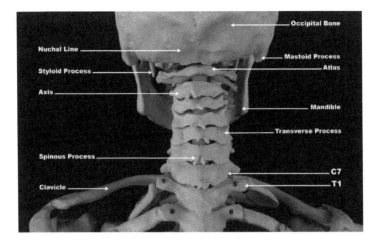

I then moved down to the shoulder and noticed a restriction in his internal rotation (see photo below), as well as a "jump off the table" reaction when I palpated the muscles of his posterior rotator cuff, which are in the back of the shoulder (teres minor, infraspinatus).

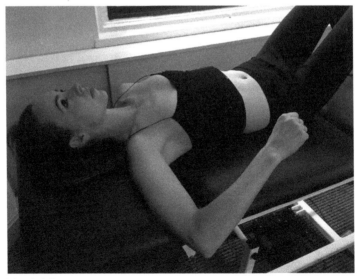

Internal rotation

Rotator Cuff Muscles

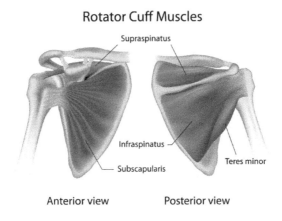

Anterior view   Posterior view

I have seen this before so it did not concern me, but putting together all of his findings with this new revelation indicated to me that the elbow was not the only problem here.

What Worked:

So where should your physiotherapist go if you present similarly? To the source(s) of the problem.

This included:

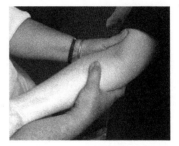

- Manual therapy to his upper neck to increase mobility, particularly to his atlas and axis

- Soft tissue release to the muscles of the upper neck and his posterior rotator cuff

Secondary treatment to the elbow included:

- Joint mobilization to the elbow joint (see inset photo)

- Modification of ergonomics at the office (As a matter of fact, I went to his office to adjust the chair, work station, and desk to make sure that was not going to continue to perpetuate the problem.)

- Soft tissue release to some of the muscles of the forearm

- Addition of eccentric[157] exercises for the wrist/elbow complex, as they are considered quite helpful for these conditions.[158,159]

---

157   Eccentric (or negative), exercise is defined as one in which there is an overall lengthening of the muscle rather than a shortening, which is concentric.

158   Stasinopoulos, D.; Manias, P., Stasinopoulou, K. "Comparing the effects of eccentric training with eccentric training and static stretching exercises in the treatment of patellar tendinopathy," Journal of Hand Therapy, Vol 26, Issue 5, 2012.

159   Tyler TF, Nicholas SJ, Schmitt BM, Mullaney M2, Hogan, DE; "Clinical outcomes of the addition of eccentrics for rehabilitation of previously failed treatments of golfers elbow," International Journal of Sports Physical Therapy, Vol 9, Iss 3: 65-70. May 2014.

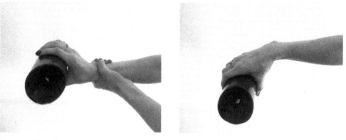

Eccentric Wrist Extension

Eccentric (or negative), exercise is defined as one in which there is an overall lengthening of the muscle rather than a shortening, which is concentric.

- We also added some stretches to normalize his shoulder internal rotation, so he did not have to compensate at this elbow anymore.

- Nerve glides for the radial and median nerves. His issue was not directly nerve related, nor was he experiencing any frank numbness or pins and needles. But when a joint gets swollen or irritated, the nerves surrounding it can get cranky. It is important to get the blood flow going again so healing can begin (see page 203 for a picture of a median nerve glide).

There are some really novel ways you can mobilize nerves here. David Butler of the Neuro Orthopedic Group (NOI) has a great video on YouTube called "Tennis Elbow-Centre Court"[160] where he shows you some great and fun ways nerves can be mobilized in different positions. After all, it has to be fun, right?

I believe the modifications made to his office set up were key, as they were really feeding into the problem. And the eccentric exercises were also paramount as well. When you have a chronic tendon issue, whether it is achilles, patella—or any tendon, for that matter, that has been subjected to constant strain or repetitive loading—the ultimate goal is eventually to remodel the tendon and allow it to adapt to load.

---

160   https://www.youtube.com/watch?v=ExaLbUdF-hw

Positive Results

Performing all of the above got him there. Elbow pain does not go away quickly, in my opinion. However, awareness of certain activities that make elbow pain worse go a long way in mitigating the morbidity associated with this condition. The patient returned to his normal gym routine and permanently added the exercises and nerve glides to his program.

Chronic pain
should have its
own diagnosis

What to Do Now

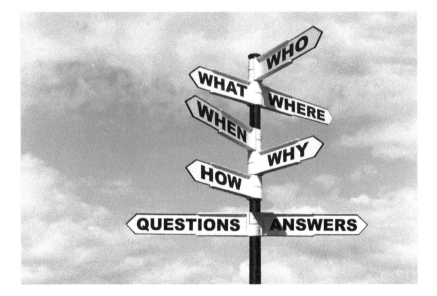

Throughout this book, I have emphasized the concept of symptom versus cause. In most cases, treating the painful part is not the same as treating the why, the origin, the root cause of your pain. In order to fully heal, you must focus on your *whole* self.

With persistent pain, pain that is not going away, you MUST consider that there could be another source to your problem.

I really like the term *healing* because, in my mind, it encompasses not just the painful part but your whole body—including your brain, your heart, and your nervous system. As I mentioned in the initial parts of this book, I have had many an injury over the years. Some went away quickly, but most did not. When you experience prolonged pain, whatever the time frame, healing seems more apropos than "fixing" or "getting rid of" it. Pain gets to you. It makes you angry, depressed, and just downright anti-social.

Many people have this limiting belief that if they do not get better, then there are no other options. That is simply NOT true. Advocate, speak up, and believe in your body's ability to heal. If you are not getting the results you want, then seek someone else out. Physical therapists are experts in movement. I would hate to see you lost to another profession. Many of my patients finally reach me after a long journey from practitioner to practitioner, with no more answers to their pain questions than when they started.

" You want someone to find the root cause of your problem, don't you? "

Make a conscious effort to find a physiotherapist who is open to looking up and down the kinetic chain to determine if there is another cause to your problem. Put your body into the hands of someone who is truly collaborative. That means they are willing to refer to an acupuncturist, a massage therapist, a Reiki Master, a nutritionist, an intuitive, a naturopath, whoever else is necessary to YOUR care.

There are many highly talented physical therapists out there who have the clinical reasoning skills, the manual skills, as well as the caring and nurturing personalities that you need. You deserve to find someone who will welcome you into their care with wide-open minds and big hearts.

You may have to pay out of pocket to get this type of care. But don't you think your health is worth it? It is all a matter of priorities. There are many people out there who won't put down one plug nickel for their care. Not because they cannot afford it, but I believe it is because they do not understand the value of going outside the traditional in network health care model. Unfortunately, with our current health care system the way it is, and insurance payment stresses as they are, oftentimes value is overlooked and lost.

With the current insurance model in the United States, I believe there is a sense of false entitlement about who should pay for health care services. Just because you have health insurance, that does not mean that all services all covered. Certainly not in this day and age. There are many progressive and innovative physical therapists out there who have opted out of the insurance model so that they can give premium (exceptional and superior) care and spend more time with their patients. What can be more important than your health? Right?

You want someone to find the root cause of your problem, don't you? Oftentimes, it really is about finding the right *person* for you. This can be a stressful experience, especially if you have been to many health care professionals. A patient of mine saw three doctors, two physical therapists, and an osteopath before she came into my office. That kind of journey knocks the stuffing out of you, raises your stress level, and makes you think that there are no answers.

The fear of the unknown can affect us in different ways. For some it causes more stress, increases the cortisol level in the blood, and creates a vicious cycle. For others, it has the opposite effect: "Thank God no one has found anything bad or sinister."

Remember, where you experience your symptom may not necessarily be the cause of your problem. Sometimes it is, but the longer you have had it, I believe it becomes secondary.

Now you are thinking, "Okay, this is all fine and good, but what do I do now?" I believe awareness and knowledge are half the battle, so to speak.

- How do I take what is incorporated in this book and apply it to myself?

- How do I find someone who can help me like this?

- What do I do if I can't find anyone?

In the first chapter of this book ("Are You Ready to Discover Why You Hurt?"), I attempt to answer questions and dispel some myths about what constitutes good physical therapy. I talk about advocating for yourself when it comes to choosing the right health care provider. Just because someone has a nice, fancy website, this does not mean they are the right person for you. Their message has to resonate. See if they have a guide or a PDF download on their site that you could read. I have one on my site called, "8 Surprising Reasons Why You Are In Pain."

There is not one person out there who has not gone down the rabbit hole of Google, looking for answers to their pain. We have all done it. I also mentioned on pages 13-14 about looking for someone through social media. That also can be quite subjective, but it is a start. If you have persistent pain, don't you want to find the right health care professional for you? It is worth spending the time to look for a good one. Re-read the first chapter of the book. At the very least, you will be armed with knowledge about the type of experience you should have when you are in good hands.

And lastly, please feel free to contact me through my website with any questions you may have. I know a lot of good physiotherapists in and out of the United States. You probably are also wondering how you can help yourself, whether you are in physical therapy or not. Our human bodies are remarkably equipped to handle many physical problems. We need to do our part to support this beautiful system.

When we are worried, anxious and in pain, our fight or flight response[161] is enhanced. Our sympathetic nervous system[162] goes into overdrive. An important system when confronted with a bear, for example. And when this system is on overdrive, our pain response is enhanced.[163]

You deserve a wonderful life. I believe that we all need different things in order for our bodies to heal. What works for someone else may not work for you. However, I believe movement is one of the foundations for your personal plan.

Movement is music for the soul. The way you move will be different from the way I move. Movement and exercise are important for healing. You can dance in your living room, jump rope, take a spin class, take a walk in the woods, or just run down the block—you get it. Movement is one prescription for persistent pain. "Motion is life."

---

161   The fight-or-flight response is a physiological reaction that occurs in response to a perceived harmful event, attack, or threat to survival.

162   The sympathetic nervous system is part of the autonomic nervous system (ANS). The sympathetic nervous system activates what is often termed the fight or flight response.

163   "Chronic Fatigue Syndrome, Irritable Bowel Syndrome, and Interstitial Cystitis: A Review of Case Control Studies." Journal of Clinical Rheumatology, Vol 20, Iss 3, 145-50: Apr 2014.

Practicing *mindfulness*[164] is also crucial. Being present can be one of the most relaxing things you can do for yourself. This helps activate the parasympathetic nervous system,[165] which is necessary to getting you back to a healthy and vibrant life. For example, Dr. John-Kabat Zinn's Mindfulness Based Stress Reduction (MSBR)[166] focuses on mindfulness interventions that improve mental and physical health. It is no secret that this type of practice helps decrease chronic pain.[167, 168]

Breathing exercises are also very helpful. If you *meditate*, then the breath work is even more enhanced and it is *mindful!* There are many different techniques out there to get you to breathe differently to achieve a quiet and relaxed mind. There are some really interesting ways breathing can help you support your musculoskeletal system via regulating the diaphragm during functional tasks.[169]

Having a *support system* is vitally important when you are dealing with persistent pain. It could be members of your family, friends—both virtual or in person. Join an online group dedicated to persistent pain. This should be an *empowering experience*—not a depressing one.

The powerful effect of community and support on pain levels is profound. Research shows that social support, perceived or actual, is associated

---

164   Mindfulness: the quality or state of being conscious or aware of something; a mental state achieved by focusing one's awareness on the present moment, while calmly acknowledging and accepting one's feelings, thoughts, and bodily sensations, used as a therapeutic technique.

165   *Parasympathetic nervous system*: Sometimes called the rest and digest system, the parasympathetic system conserves energy as it slows the heart rate, increases intestinal and gland activity, and relaxes sphincter muscles in the gastrointestinal tract.

166   "Jon Kabat-Zinn: Defining Mindfulness." Jan 11, 2016: http://www.mindful.org/jon-kabat-zinn-defining-mindfulness/

167   Baer, Ruth A. Mindfulness-Based Treatment Approaches: Clinician's Guide to Evidence Base and Applications. Academic Press: 2015.

168   Garland, Eric L; Manusov, Eron G; Froelinger, Brett; Kelly, Amber; Williams, Jaclyn M; Howard, Matthew O. "Mindfulness-oriented recovery enhancement for chronic pain and prescription opioid misuse: Results from an early-stage randomized controlled trial." Journal of Consulting and Clinical Psychology, Vol 82, Iss 3. Jun 2014, 448-459.

169   Paed, Pavel Kolaf; Sulc, Jan; Kynci, Martin; Sanda, Jan; Cakrt, Ondfej; Andel, Ross; Kumagim Kathryn; Kobesova, Alena. "Postural Function of the Diaphragm in Persons With and Without Chronic Low-back Pain." Journal of Orthopaedic & Sports Physical Therapy, Vol 42, Iss 4, 2012.

with reduced pain perception across several health conditions.[170] I will go so far as to say that loneliness should be considered a public health issue.[171] It certainly has an effect on pain. Loneliness kills more people than smoking and alcoholism. Think about that for a second. Let that one sink in.

> " In his book, Loneliness, John Cacioppo, a psychologist at the University of Chicago, says that the pain of loneliness is akin to physical pain. "

When you have persistent pain, feeling alone and unsupported affects you in a way that may prevent you from moving forward in your healing journey. In a research report published in 2013, it is shown that the pain, depression, and fatigue symptom cluster is an important health concern. Loneliness is a common risk factor for these symptoms.[172,173]

As a matter of fact, loneliness has around twice the impact on an early death as obesity. TWICE THE RISK.

In his book, *Loneliness*, John Cacioppo, a psychologist at the University of Chicago, says that the pain of loneliness is akin to physical pain.[174]

Get in touch with your *spirituality*. This means letting go of who you think you are and becoming your true authentic self. Demands imposed upon us during everyday life force us to choose between ourselves and something or someone else. More often than not, we put ourselves last. This type of behaviour is not helpful in getting rid of persistent pain. Seek wisdom and guidance from others. Get *creative*—try a therapeutic coloring

---

170   Sarason, IG; Sarason, BR; Shearin, EN; Pierce, GR. "A brief measure of support: Practical and theoretical implications." Journal of Social and Personal Relationships, Vol 4, Iss 4, 497-510: 1987.

171   Lissa Rankin Ted Talk: https://www.youtube.com/watch?v=s2hLhWSlOl0

172   Jaremka, Lisa M; Fagundes, Christopher P; Glaser, Ronald; Bennett, Jeanette M; Malarkey, William B; Kiecolt-Glaser, Janice K. "Loneliness Predicts Pain, Depression, and Fatigue: Understanding the Role of Immune Dysregulation." Psychoneuroendocrinology, Vol 38, Iss 8: Aug 2013.

173   Wolf, Laurie Dempsey; Davis, Mary C. "Loneliness, Daily Pain, and Perceptions of Interpersonal events in Adults with Fibromyalgia." Health Psychology, Vol 33, Iss 9, 929-937: Sept 2014.

174   Cacioppo, John. Patrick, William. Loneliness, Human Nature, and the Need for Social Connection. W. W. Norton & Company, 2008.

book. They are very popular and can help you calm your nervous system.

If you have dropped your favorite exercise practice, find ways to get involved again, even if it is for five to ten minutes. It is a start. I mentioned in another chapter about *graded exposure to exercise and graded motor imagery* (see page 192), that this is an important component to helping you move better again. It is not a boom-or-bust scenario. You feel good and go all out and then the next day, you can't move! It is about taking small steps and thinking about the bigger picture or bigger vision for your body and your health. People who want quick results immediately almost never look at the big picture scenario.

Other options can include *Emotional Freedom Technique* (**EFT**) **or** *"tapping."* This is a healing modality that combines Ancient Chinese acupressure and modern psychology. I have not had firsthand experience with this, but I believe it is worth exploring. For more information, go to www.thetappingsolution.com.

Also, do not underestimate the power of certain foods on chronic pain. Seek out the *advice of a nutritionist or registered dietician.* I have many patients who, when they add and eliminate certain foods from their diet, they feel better.

Pain can be inevitable but suffering is optional.[175]

Healing is a journey that is comprised of many paths. Facing cognitive and emotional issues head-on is an important path in that journey. If you feel that you will never get better, then you will never get better. Confronting this barrier must be addressed. As I have mentioned previously, having your pain explained to you can be very therapeutic. Getting a better understanding behind all the workings of your brain and its role in pain behaviour is crucial. If you still feel that the source of your low-back pain is your back, and you are adamant in that belief, but the physical therapy evaluation reveals that it is your hip, then you will not fully recover. If you are not open to the fact that your hip is the prime cause, then you are doing yourself a huge disservice.

---

175   Lissa Rankin, Mind Over Medicine: Scientific Proof That You Can Heal Yourself. Hay House, Inc: 2013.

Movement is life.

As I was writing this book, images of both my mother and father were ingrained in my mind. Their values are firmly rooted in how I face the world on a daily basis. My mother suffered a horrific motor vehicle accident and was rendered immobile without the ability to speak or walk. I saw her courage, compassion, and determination in the face of all odds. And my father—my companion on our glorious ascent of Mt. Kiliman-jaro—was always prodding me to do my best. Then one day a fall rendered him almost immobile. I am grateful every day I get up and put one foot in front of the other, even if it *hurts*.

This puts a lot into perspective when we do lose our ability to move, let alone move well. Movement means different things for different people. But I do believe that we have the inherent capacity to intuitively find ways to move when we are hurting and unable to move. That is the beauty of the human body.

Maybe it starts with a breath and then a gentle movement of the legs or a wiggling of the toe and fingers. Or maybe we visualize and imagine our painful part moving gracefully and pain-free.[176] Whatever method or modality we choose to embrace as we face our pain issues, it is imperative that we seek the guidance of an expert along the way.

After reading this book, you should feel empowered in the knowledge that if you have not gotten the results you have wanted, then there is hope. Please seek out the services of a physical therapist and be open and truth-ful with yourself and them. If that person is not willing to have another dialogue with you about the possibility as to other causes to your problem, then you should end that relationship and move on. Lesson learned.

Finding a physical therapist who thinks out of the box and embraces a whole body approach to assessment and treatment is crucial.

---

176   Wand BM; Tullock, VM; George, PJ; Smith, AG; Goucke, R; O'Connell, NE; Moseley, GL. "Seeing It Helps: Movement-Related Back Pain Is Reduced by Visualization of the Back During Movement." Clinical Journal of Pain, Vol 28, Iss 7, 602-608: Sept 2012.

I hope I have equipped you with the knowledge about your body and how you move so that you can take that to a physical therapist and be more well-informed.

Thank you for reading my book!

Remember, your life need not be controlled or defined by pain.

About the Author

Erica Meloe is a board certified physiotherapist and co-owner of Velocity Physiotherapy, a private practice in NYC. After a decade solving financial puzzles on Wall Street, Erica took her MBA and her problem-solving skills into the clinic. She specializes in treating patients with persistent unsolved pain and her mission is to raise awareness of the physical therapy profession to a level like no other.

Erica is co-host of the podcast "Tough To Treat: A physiotherapist's guide to managing those complex patients." She is also a thought leader in the profession and helps her patients, as well as her colleagues, empower themselves to lead and live with purpose.

Erica has also been featured in Forbes, BBC, Women's Day, Better Homes and Gardens, Muscle and Fitness Hers, and Health Magazine. She is also co-host of the Women In PT Summit, held annually in NYC.

To book an appointment with her in person, or from anywhere in the world, contact her at erica@ericameloe.com.

CPSIA information can be obtained
at www.ICGtesting.com
Printed in the USA
LVHW070030141220
674072LV00022B/2355

9 780998 993904